Breastfeeding the Brave

A practical guide for health and
lactation professionals supporting families of
medically complex infants and children in the paediatric setting.

Breastfeeding the Brave: A practical guide for health and lactation professionals supporting families of medically complex infants and children in the paediatric setting.

First published in the UK by Thought Rebellion Limited 2022

ISBN 978-1-7396929-3-3

Also available as an ebook

Proofread by Jules Wraith

Cover design and all artwork: Leanne Pearce

A catalogue record for this book is available from the British Library.

Contents

This book is dedicated to
the children and families everywhere
who are fighting serious childhood illness.

#BreastfeedingTheBrave

Acknowledgements

There are numerous people to whom I am indebted and without whom not only would I have not written this book, but I also would not be the practitioner I am.

I must acknowledge the stream of incredible teachers I have had as a paediatric nurse, public health nurse, IBCLC and newbie researcher. For over twenty years I have been privileged to have learned from world-class lecturers and clinical specialists at undergraduate and postgraduate level. Latterly I am particularly indebted to Professor Amy Brown whose friendship and exhaustive knowledge of breastfeeding research has been a huge source of support and motivation.

I also have a really cool friend list which includes academics, clinicians, specialists and artists who over the years have been generous with their friendship and knowledge. I must specifically mention Helen Calvert, Sarah Edney-Dutton, Carmelle Gentle, Dr Ilana Levene, Becks Lewis, Dr Natalie Shenker, Amanda Smith, Dr Vicky Thomas, Imogen Unger, Lauren Wong and Stacey Zimmels as well as innumerable clinicians who have all been gracious with their time and expertise. Leanne Pearce's incredible artwork is stunning, and the book would be far less impactful without her beautiful and moving portraits of the families depicted.

I probably would not have written this book at all if I had not been the breastfeeding mother of children who have had more than their fair share of medical complexity. I'd like to thank Lizzy and Filly for showing me how to parent during serious and life-threatening illness, and for maintaining their sense of humour throughout some pretty awful times. I'd also be nowhere without the support of my husband Tim and my extended family and friends who provided love, meals, flowers and shoulders to cry on during some scary moments.

Finally, this book would be nothing without the extraordinary generosity of the families who have shaped it. I am beyond grateful to the members of the Breastfeeding the Brave group, my research participants and the clients I have supported over many years. Thank you for bravely sharing your stories and stunning photos with me in the hope that they make a positive impact on someone else's journey.

Abbreviations

I sometimes forget that not everyone speaks fluent 'Hospital', and that not everyone works in the UK. I have tried throughout to explain abbreviations and terms, but in case you need a reminder, here are some very common abbreviations I have referred to.

BFC	Breastfeeding Counsellor
BFHI	Baby Friendly Hospital Initiative
BFI	Baby Friendly Initiative
CICU	Cardiac Intensive Care Unit
CPAP	Continuous Positive Airway Pressure
ECMO	Extracorporeal Membrane Oxygenation
ED	Emergency Department
FCC	Family Centred Care
GMC	General Medical Council
GP	General Practitioner (Family doctor)
HDU	High Dependency Unit
HFNC	High Flow Nasal Cannula
HFOV	High-Frequency Oscillatory Ventilation
HV	Health Visitor
IBCLC	International Board Certified Lactation Consultant
IV	Intravenous
LP	Lumbar Puncture
MDT	Multidisciplinary Team
NG	Nasogastric
NICU	Neonatal Intensive Care Unit
NMC	Nursing and Midwifery Council
NNU	Neonatal Unit
NNS	Non-Nutritive sucking
PEG	Percutaneous Endoscopic Gastrostomy
PICU	Paediatric Intensive Care Unit
PS	Peer Supporter
SLT	Speech and Language Therapist
TPN	Total Parenteral Nutrition

Introduction

Welcome! Whether this is the first book you've ever read on breastfeeding, or you have a fully loaded infant feeding shelf, I'm glad you have this in your hands. This is a subject close to my heart, and before we get going I'll share with you why I'm so passionate about supporting families of sick children to breastfeed, and why I feel so strongly that this is a unique population that deserves a book all to itself.

I have been supporting sick children for twenty years as a paediatric nurse and in various other roles. I've been an International Board Certified Lactation Consultant (IBCLC) since 2011 and have dedicated my career to supporting families with breastfeeding. I am also the mother of a sepsis and childhood cancer survivor, who was breastfed throughout 26 months of treatment until she was almost six years old.

In 2019 I started working on my PhD, exploring the challenges of breastfeeding medically complex infants and children, as well as supporting their families, and the staff caring for them. Alongside the importance of breastfeeding and breast milk to families, one of the main themes that has emerged from my research is the gap in training for this important patient group.

I am privileged to know and support hundreds of inspiring parents who are breastfeeding their children through extraordinarily difficult challenges. Their perseverance and commitment inspire me every day, but so do their challenges. For every parent who has endured and persisted, many more have been let down and their efforts undermined.

I have been asking these families about their experiences for a few years, gathering their responses and using this data to interrogate the literature that we have available about breastfeeding medically complex children. I have organised polls, listened to their stories, undertaken a systematic review, and conducted two research studies - one of health professionals, the other of parent experiences. All the anecdotal, informal and published literature I can find has been used throughout this book to strengthen the evidence and rationale for considering these children as a unique population.

In sharing many of these stories, as well as information and tools, my hope is that we can strive to do better for these families.

My story

Rather unusually for a lactation advocate, my interest in breastfeeding predated my own children by at least eight years. I first became captivated by this topic during my paediatric nursing training. I qualified as a nurse in 2004 and immediately noticed that almost all of my patients were under the age of two years, and therefore the vast majority of them were milk-fed to a greater or lesser extent. Relatively few of my patients were breastfed, but when they were, there existed a tension between those providing support for infant feeding choices and those providing clinical care.

I noticed repeatedly that parents were often advised to express milk rather than directly breastfeed, so that volumes could be measured accurately. Frequently parents were also advised to supplement breastfeeding with infant formula, even when there were no obvious concerns about milk supply or weight gain. There seemed to be little understanding of how breastfeeding and lactation works, and little interest in supporting parents to meet their personal feeding goals or overcome breastfeeding problems. Rather, bottle and formula feeding were all too often presented as the solution to *any* breastfeeding issues.

Although there were some outstanding exceptions, many of my nursing and medical colleagues did not seem able or willing to support parents with breastfeeding if indeed that was their choice. This was partly because there was very little training on offer, and partly because many of them did not feel it was within their job remit. Some of them carried their own sadness, baggage or misconceptions from personal feeding experiences into their role. As far as some of my colleagues were concerned, while nutrition was an important part of illness management and recovery, the nuances of that nutrition were deemed less significant than clinical care and counting calories.

In common with many of my colleagues, I had received just two hours of training in infant feeding as part of my undergraduate degree. This covered some of the 'benefits of breastfeeding' and some basic positioning tips, and I was considered lucky to have had that. I frequently overheard advice being given that was not evidence-based, and as I began to study in my own time I realised how much professionals in paediatrics did *not* know. The gap became painfully evident, especially when I compared it to my student experiences rotating through neonatal intensive care and health visiting.

Another early observation was the fact that I could not (and did not want to) separate caring for a breastfeeding mother and her sick child. I often cared for mothers of infants less than two weeks old and quickly accepted that the two could not be considered separate entities. Yet the systems and structures were not set up to facilitate this – for example, bedsharing was frowned upon. There also did not seem to be much consideration for how paediatric nurses with no adult nursing or midwifery training should care for a mother who has recently given birth, besides directing her back to her midwife – which would mean sending her to another ward or department, without her baby. It was all very unsatisfactory and felt disjointed.

I still remember the baby that changed everything for me. He's all grown up now and wouldn't know me if he bumped into me in the street. But he and his mother are responsible for being the fork in the road of my career. Most people fall into lactation advocacy and support after the experience of breastfeeding their own children, which is a wonderful thing - but that's not what happened to me.

I was a newly minted paediatric nurse, wearing my shiny and hard-earned Florence Nightingale School of Nursing and Midwifery badge from Kings College with pride. I was acutely aware that I knew nothing really, about anything at all. However, I was searching for something to get my teeth stuck into. My peers were busy doing cardiac specialist nurse training or developing passions for trauma or intensive care. Exciting, adrenaline-fuelled sub-specialities. But none of the clinical specialties I was exposed to held my gaze – not liver transplant, intensive care, oncology, surgery, or anything else. So I waited it out rather impatiently on a general paediatric ward, hoping that the future would declare itself, or I'd find a way out of nursing – being honest, I didn't really mind which.

Then, one night shift, a mother walked slowly and laboriously up the ward towards me. Every step was measured and careful - a wrong move provoked a visible cringe. The emergency department (ED) nurse ahead of her wheeled a bassinet containing this woman's 3-day-old bright yellow (he was significantly jaundiced and was being admitted for phototherapy) baby son whose bilirubin level was impressive. A porter trailed behind carrying overnight bags. I can't explain what happened logically or rationally, but my heart seemed to move in my chest. I was only 22 years old, not a mother myself and yet I could feel that this mother and her son needed care that supported them *both*. Of course I set up the double phototherapy that this little one needed. Of course I did my admission paperwork like all good nurses should do (this was in the dark ages when nursing records were not electronic dear friends). But I also helped that sore and bewildered mother to set up her breast pump, get comfortable (ish), and begin to trust me. Something happened that night, and all I can say is that I became a breastfeeding advocate for life. Back then I probably didn't do a very good job of explaining how to use the breast pump. I cringe at how little I knew about hand expressing at the time. But I made that mother laugh, and cry happy tears - she relaxed, and the milk came. Her baby went back to her breast. I was hooked. I realised that the paediatric ward was not an ideal place to have a breastfeeding crisis, but making paediatrics better was part of making breastfeeding better – and perhaps vice versa.

We will return to this topic, but Baby Friendly Initiative (BFI) standards (a set of standards which exist to protect and support breastfeeding) apply to many maternity settings, neonatal wards, health visiting teams, children's centres and even some universities. Not paediatrics. This is a grave mistake. This means that children from as young as one or two days old might be admitted to an environment in which breastfeeding training is not embedded, and the staff not invested. Perhaps you might think that it is all so obvious that we can just get on with it. However, the problem is that if there is no policy, research or standard training requirement, it does not get prioritised. Breastfeeding joins the back of the (very long) queue and any proposed change or policy implementation falls flat when someone asks the fatal question - where is the evidence? It certainly might feel like a no-brainer to those of us in the know but in an evidence-based environment, not having research to back up your recommendations means that it's basically not going to happen.

Family centred care (FCC) was and remains a key principle of caring for children in hospital, and it seemed particularly relevant when sick children were having breastfeeding difficulties. However, when it came to these real-world situations, the theory and practice did not always gel. Keeping families together, valuing parents as partners in care, upholding and respecting the customs and traditions of families, sharing responsibility and valuing their wisdom and opinion are all important to the concept of FCC (Mikkelsen and Frederiksen, 2011; Dennis et al, 2017). I felt that these concepts applied perfectly to protecting a parent's choice to breastfeed and yet this didn't seem to be universally valued in the paediatric setting.

Family centred care, lactation and paediatrics are so obviously, naturally, intricately woven and yet not well integrated. I still remember the 'old-school' ward sister who, over a decade ago said to me *'I'm all for family centred care, but when it comes to critical care, it has to take a back seat'*. I feel like that sentence lit a fire in me, and ever since I've been determined to prove her wrong.

I worked for a few years as the regional FCC coordinator for a large perinatal network covering four neonatal units, including a tertiary referral centre. The difference between the neonatal and paediatric settings in terms of the wide acceptance of breastfeeding as the biological norm in the former was stark. Breastfeeding was not only accepted, it was expected and valued as part of the immunological, developmental and emotional support for extremely preterm neonates, as well as critically unstable term neonates with congenital anomalies and other medical complexities. Donor human milk was viewed by some as medicine in the neonatal unit (NNU), whereas on the paediatric ward you'd have thought I was suggesting that we feed our little patients dirty dishwater. I wondered over and over again why paediatrics had such a different culture.

After a few years within the in-patient paediatric and neonatal setting, I moved into the community, and trained as a health visitor (HV). I then became more exposed to the challenges of infant feeding within the context of public health nursing. I sub-specialised in lactation and qualified as an International Board Certified Lactation Consultant (IBCLC) in 2011. I became increasingly aware of the gap between clinical paediatrics and optimal breastfeeding support, noticing that many nonclinical lactation supporters and indeed health visitors with an adult nursing or direct entry midwifery background have limited knowledge of how to support very sick children. Equally, most paediatric clinicians have limited knowledge of how to support lactation. In my experience, it is clear that very few professionals have dual skill sets in paediatric clinical care *and* lactation (Hookway, 2020). Even during my health visitor training,

I received no mandatory training in infant feeding. Breastfeeding training was only made available if the health visiting team was pursuing baby-friendly accreditation. Even then, the instruction received was partially dependent on the skills of the Infant Feeding Lead, which was one reason I took up this post after a few years in general health visiting.

This journey became much more personal when my second breastfed child, Filly, became critically sick with sepsis at the age of three and was subsequently diagnosed with acute lymphoblastic leukaemia (ALL). We breastfed through 26 months of chemotherapy, thousands of painful procedures and countless hospital admissions, and received little to no encouragement for breastfeeding through our journey. I perhaps didn't need breastfeeding support from the healthcare professionals, and frankly would have continued anyway. However, it did make me reflect that had I not been an experienced IBCLC and breastfeeding advocate, I might have stopped breastfeeding during one of our many feeding, medication or weight hurdles along the way.

There isn't much that is positive about having a child who has survived not one, but two life-threatening conditions, except perhaps that it gave me a much-needed nudge to formalise the support I had been quietly offering families for many years. I realised how urgently parents of breastfed sick children needed bespoke support, and also how few professionals are well-positioned, and suitably educated to provide it.

On completion of Filly's treatment, when our personal trauma felt less raw, I established the Breastfeeding the Brave project – which started as a small online Facebook support group for other mothers breastfeeding through serious, chronic, life-threatening, critical, or palliative illness. While most people at that time knew me for the responsive sleep advocacy and support I provide, I had made no secret of our cancer journey; many people reached out to me during Filly's treatment, keen to hear how I had managed to breastfeed through childhood cancer. The group now has several hundred members all regularly sharing challenges, inspiration, experiences and support with each other. I have informally acted as an advocate for many of them who have received opposition to continuing to breastfeed their very sick children. As awareness has grown of the gap in knowledge and support within paediatrics, many professionals have also joined the group in an effort to learn. Thus, my personal journey has collided with my IBCLC skill set, teaching experience, research and clinical paediatric nursing experience.

Throughout the last twenty years of clinical nursing experience, providing specialised lactation support on the paediatric ward, neonatal unit, in health visiting roles and infant feeding lead roles, I have drawn on my IBCLC and nursing training, skills and knowledge. I have also been frustrated at how little coverage is given to supporting sick children in currently available training and have had to merge my nursing and lactation skills many times to create a 'mash-up' of suggestions. I have observed how breastfeeding mother-child dyads are cared for within multiple settings, including a personal one. I see the need for a closing of the gulf between clinical paediatrics and infant feeding support, and hope that my research, the training that I offer, and this book can go some way to filling the space between two, so far, fairly distinct disciplines.

It has been my experience over the years that people are most transformed by hearing the stories of those who are the main characters. I consider myself extraordinarily privileged to be acquainted with many incredible parents who were part of the original Breastfeeding the Brave group. Their stories, and the stories of their children inspire me every day to continue to work hard to make breastfeeding in paediatrics better. Several of them graciously agreed to allow me to publish their story in this book, with the hope of making things better for other parents in the future. Even more amazingly, the wonderfully talented Leanne Pearce agreed to immortalise them in oil. I hope their stories and portraits bring these issues to life for you.

Leanne is a portrait artist working and living in the Northeast of England. She is motivated by making purposeful work, and her most recent collections include 'Breastfeed - Portraits with Purpose' and 'Breastfeeding the Brave'. Leanne has exhibited her artwork throughout the UK in group and solo exhibitions at universities, galleries, hospitals and public spaces. Her work also resides in private collections in the US and Australia.

She has appeared twice as a contestant on Sky Arts Portrait Artist of the Year and gained a place in the national semi-finals of the

ITV show 'A Brush With Fame' in which she painted a whole host of celebrities including Tanni Grey-Thompson and Paul Nicholas.

Leanne is a mother of two daughters. She is also an accredited Breastfeeding Peer Supporter. She feels passionately about breastfeeding and supporting mothers through their time breastfeeding. Her ambition is to educate as an activist but always display compassion and understanding through her artwork.

"I indulge my passion for painting most days and I am motivated by making artwork which I deem to be useful and significant, in work I refer to as 'Portraits with Purpose'. I want to reveal truths and a deeper understanding of human experiences, of motherhood, women's work and in particular highlighting and celebrating breastfeeding. I have been creating portraiture with breastfeeding at the forefront since having my own children. No better medium than large scale portraits of breastfeeding mothers to celebrate women's work, of which I created 20 paintings in a series titled 'Breastfeed'. It is significant to me to show fragility, bravery, humanity, love and care in intense, realistic paintings.

My artwork offers complex and emotional viewpoints, triggering questioning and thought. Every detail is painstakingly tended to through oil paint and tiny brushes as if caring for the people I paint. I am intrigued by the glint in the eye, the tilt of the head, the fold of the fabric and the relationships in the artwork. In 'Breastfeeding the Brave' I am also exploring the setting and context, something new for me, the wires and tubes that channel liquids and air, the monitors that register heart rates and the hand pump for breath; juxtaposing medical intervention against human life."

Leanne Pearce

Acknowledging the many distinct areas of specialism and expertise

I'm aware that the readers of this book will have a huge range of experience, training and backgrounds. Some of you will be highly experienced at supporting lactation, and yet have very little or no health professional qualifications or clinical background. Others of you will be highly proficient at managing the care of critically sick children, but have little to no experience, or training in lactation. A rare few of you may have skills in both areas. I'm also aware that some of you may not be familiar with either topic, or perhaps picked up this book out of sheer curiosity or because of the artwork! Please take what you need from this book, and while some areas might feel more or less familiar depending on where your primary skill set lies, I hope you find it helpful to view this through a different lens.

I'm acutely conscious that many committed individuals have been tirelessly working in this area for many years, and we all stand on their shoulders. Much of the research that exists does not apply directly to sick older children or nursing toddlers, but we can borrow and adapt it. Many people have developed ways to improve care for this population group, and where possible, I have tried to find this unpublished work which is based on the work of very experienced colleagues.

Whether clinical care or lactation support is your stronger area, this book is designed to bridge two, so far, fairly distinct areas of specialism for the purpose of improving care for families. Whatever your own journey into health or lactation care, I want to thank you personally, as a mother, IBCLC, and nurse for making the time to read this.

Some notes about content and language

Before we get going in earnest, it's probably an obvious point but in this book, I will be discussing stories and scenarios of very sick children. Many of the families I have met, spoken with, interviewed and got to know have endured trauma, very difficult and long treatments and some have suffered bereavement. Some of you will be experienced at handling this, and others may not. Can I encourage you to talk to someone if you find any of the information in this book triggering or upsetting? Find a trusted friend, colleague or ally with whom you can debrief.

Secondly, I am committed in my practice to using inclusive terms and additive language wherever possible, such as breast and chestfeeding, human milk, mothers, fathers, parents and lactation (Zimman, 2017; Dinour, 2019). This is not to erase anyone, but simply to include those who do not feel represented by the words mother, breast or woman. I also acknowledge that some people have suffered trauma, abuse or rape, and sometimes for these reasons prefer not to use the word breast. I'm conscious that use of language, whether inclusive or gender normative, tends to divide opinion and occasionally become the subject of heated debate. My personal take with this is that while it does not affect *my* mental health to include additional words, or change the words around from time to time, it may seriously negatively affect someone *else's* mental health if I omit those words. I have long since committed to choosing an approach that is compassionate and understanding, while at the same time recognising that these issues are complex and sometimes deeply personal and emotive.

I would rather be criticised for who I include, than for who I exclude.

However, *most* of the parents I have supported over the years have identified as mothers, so you will hear me use that word most often. Having said that, I have also supported lactating non-binary, trans and queer parents and professionals and I acknowledge and honour them as well. This is an important topic and a unique book, and I don't wish the language to distract from its clinical importance. Therefore, throughout the book, for ease of reading I tend to use the words 'mother' and 'breastfeeding', but please know that I respect and value the words you prefer to use.

Finally, I want to acknowledge that we all bring different experiences of feeding with us. I want you to know that I understand that this is an emotive issue, and many people feel disappointed, let down or hurt by their experiences with feeding their own babies. I urge you to seek debrief support with a breastfeeding counsellor, psychologist or IBCLC if you find it hard to reconcile your own experiences with the need to support other families.

As you make your way through this book, I will be inviting you to consider aspects of practice and asking questions at the end of each chapter to help you reflect. Write down your questions as you go along and note any areas where you feel you may need more support, training, supervision or information. This is a relatively unresearched breastfeeding specialty and there are many unanswered questions. I would consider it a success if reading this provokes further lines of enquiry and curiosity.

We will be covering:

- How infant feeding works, including the mechanism of feeding, milk production, and human milk specificity.
- How to support optimal breastfeeding, including which professionals provide support, and the interventions known to help.
- The importance and meaning of breastfeeding sick and complex children to families.
- The current gaps in policy and learning provision.
- Some understanding of how supporting medically complex children differs from healthy children, or those in the neonatal setting.
- The importance of FCC, and what this means as a lived reality.
- Some ideas for how to work with the multidisciplinary team (the many different professionals who come into contact with sick children as part of their care – for example, nurses, doctors, speech and language therapists, dietitians and so on) to co-create practical feeding plans with families.
- Helping you to reflect on how to balance feeding goals with clinical priorities.
- Additional skills that may be necessary to support certain groups of children.

A note on 'bravery'

This book shares its name with the name of the group I started a few years ago. A few people have questioned the use of the word 'brave', pointing out that children who are sick have no choice but to endure their treatment, and the word bravery could imply that they do this willingly, sacrificially, or uncomplainingly. Bravery has many connotations and assumptions – several of which are unhelpful. I know this very well from a personal perspective. When Filly was diagnosed with cancer, she initially tolerated central line accesses with apparent ease. She barely flinched, and the nurses used to tell her how 'brave' she was. She earned a reputation for being 'easy'. After about 6 months of that, it was like she had decided she'd had enough of being 'brave', if brave meant being quiet and still, and acting like it didn't hurt and that it was all ok.

She yelled and fought and wouldn't be still. We negotiated and begged and bribed and gave warning and didn't give warning, and let her make some of the choices and call some of the shots. Nothing 'worked'. And then I decided it was the definition of bravery that was the problem. Bravery is not putting on a smile when you feel like shouting. It is not staying still and quiet and acting like it doesn't matter or it doesn't hurt, or that you don't hate every second of it.

Bravery is sometimes a loud, roaring thing.

Bravery complains and fights back. Bravery is not about being tough, but about being soft and human and vulnerable and letting that show. Breastfeeding the Brave was very much written from this perspective of the concept of bravery, not some sanitised version that has everyone smiling cheerfully and maintaining a stiff upper lip. Of course, when I speak of bravery, I am also referring to the stoicism, resilience and courage of the mothers, fathers, parents and partners, siblings, grandparents and wider family and friends who also must endure the challenges of illness and medical complexity. Bravery also applies to the health and lactation professionals who sometimes have to have difficult conversations and undertake procedures they wish they didn't need to.

Why this work is important

In late 2020, as part of my PhD, I invited paediatric health care professionals in the UK to take part in a survey that sought to discover attitudes, challenges and barriers regarding lactation support in the paediatric setting. Recognising that many professionals provide care to paediatric patients outside of the paediatric ward – for example paediatric surgery and the emergency department - participation was invited from anyone caring for children in hospital. Nearly 500 professionals responded to the survey, about half of whom were paediatric nurses, and about 150 were doctors of various training grades and levels of experience. I also had several responses from allied health professionals such as physiotherapists, speech and language therapists and dietitians.

Half of those surveyed did not feel confident or experienced enough to support parents with lactation challenges, and very few had extensive breastfeeding or lactation training. Only a handful were qualified to IBCLC or breastfeeding counsellor level. The vast majority of participants said that their knowledge came from their own experiences. Most of them said that they had *no* breastfeeding training as part of their initial undergraduate training and those who *had* received training had, on the whole, received only one to two hours. Almost all of them felt that their training had not equipped them to be able to support their patients in the paediatric setting, and most felt they needed or would benefit from training. All but a handful of them felt that different skills are needed to support children in paediatrics.

What health professionals want to know

When I broke down exactly what health professionals wanted to know, and where the problems were, three quarters felt that during an average shift there was not enough support for families, and that the biggest barrier to staff being able to support parents was lack of knowledge. Several of the professionals surveyed held specialist feeding roles, ran feeding clinics or had some kind of additional recognized responsibility for infant feeding. However, many of them did not feel confident about basic areas such as assessing the effectiveness of milk transfer. The knowledge gaps identified by staff included improving latch to reduce nipple pain, identifying poor milk transfer, supporting common breastfeeding challenges, protecting and increasing milk supply, as well as promoting the benefits of non-nutritive suckling. Most professionals also reported that they did not feel confident supporting more complex cases – such as babies and children with higher calorie needs, low tone, orofacial anomalies, and returning to direct breastfeeding after enteral feeding. Most of the professionals felt that specialised breastfeeding training is needed to support professionals who are caring for sick children - and I wholeheartedly agree.

To that end, in this book:

- I will review how breastfeeding works. I'll cover the definitions and prevalence of illness and medical complexity, and use this, with the knowledge of infant feeding fundamental skills to help you understand why breastfeeding medically complex children is harder.

- I will share some of my research into the challenges of feeding sick children and how we can create a better environment for families facing these challenges as well as how to preserve milk supply.

- I will also explore the world of equipment and skills necessary to support these families.

- I am also going to cover several specific clinical situations that may require specialised knowledge and skills.

- Finally, I will end by considering how to weave family-centred care into everyday practice, and challenge some commonly held beliefs that might still exist. Throughout the book, I will provide case studies and examples to help you translate theory into practice.

What I will *not* be covering

In the interest of providing information that is implementable and succinct, I have left out certain information that cannot be covered within the scope of this book. That includes specific clinical details about certain conditions, and management guidelines for each condition. What is not necessarily helpful is for staff to have to search for specific guidelines on each condition. Therefore, to make this information as user-friendly as possible to busy staff, I have grouped challenges - where possible - by their impact on lactation and breastfeeding. For example, rather than have a specific guideline for diabetes, cystic fibrosis, heart defect, cancer and bronchiolitis, I have grouped strategies and resources more generally where possible – for example low tone, high calorie need, sleepiness and fasting times. Some specific conditions do require some nuance and I have briefly covered those in Chapter 9.

I am also frequently asked about supporting breastfeeding in parents who are sick. This is an entirely different (and very important) area of support, and I will not specifically be covering it, though many of the principles covered will apply to sick mothers who are lactating as well. Some good resources for medications in lactation can be found in the appendix, including Wendy Jones' helpful book *Breastfeeding and Medication* (2013), and the Breastfeeding Network *Drugs in Breastfeeding* information sheets.

Chapter 1

Why Breastfeeding Matters

We have to begin by understanding that breastfeeding is the biologically normal and expected way to feed infants and children for the first two years of life and beyond. This sometimes feels uncomfortable to hear and is not intended to represent a moral or socially deterministic view. However, all mammals make species-specific milk for their young, and while this is not a 100% perfect system, it is incontestable that this is the biological standard. The World Health Organisation recommends exclusive breastfeeding for six months, and then alongside solid family foods for two years or beyond (WHO, 2014). Some studies suggest that the normal duration of breastfeeding is anywhere from two to seven years (Dettwyler, 2004), and anecdotal data supports this.

However, there is sometimes a misunderstanding about the word 'normal' or 'natural'. Just because something is normal, does not necessarily make it easy. In fact, this can feel dismissive or even triggering for many people. I'm sure many of you have first-hand experience of either going through your own challenges, or supporting families, clients, patients or friends with theirs. Breastfeeding is not easy. Just like the natural behaviour of walking is a learned skill, so too is breastfeeding. We are social beings, and we learn many skills by watching others. The fewer people we see breastfeeding, and meeting their feeding goals, the harder it is to learn from others. We also have good instincts, but this can become drowned out by too many conflicting opinions, or erroneous information. Sometimes in order to hear our instinct, we have to learn to silence the noise.

Challenges are common, even among low-risk mother and baby dyads. Perceptions of low milk supply, nipple pain, excessive infant weight loss and unrealistic expectations of infant behaviour make this normal behaviour much more challenging, and lead to many people stopping breastfeeding before they planned to. As Professor Amy Brown (2018) has written about, stopping breastfeeding before parents feel ready can lead to feelings of grief, sadness, depression, and in some cases, trauma.

When we speak about promoting breastfeeding support, we are not talking about *forcing* parents to breastfeed against their will. As a lactation advocate, it is not my job to impose my opinions and goals on other parents. Feeding goals are intensely personal and the job of a lactation supporter is to facilitate the achievement of those personal goals whether the mother or parent's goal is to breastfeed for two days, two weeks, two months, two years or more (Fahlquist et al, 2016). A self-defined feeding goal may also include exclusive expressing, holding in arms while tube feeding, or combination feeding. Whatever a mother/parent's goal is, in order to achieve it, they need accurate information, realistic expectations and excellent health, lactation and social support.

The biological specificity and public health importance of human milk

Not forgetting the individuality of infant feeding decision-making, when we look at the bigger picture, breastfeeding is important for individuals, communities, wider public health outcomes and economies. Ensuring that as many children as possible are exclusively breastfed for the first six months of life and then alongside appropriate introduction of complementary foods until the age of two years or beyond would prevent 800,000 deaths in children under five per year globally (Holla-Bhar et al, 2015). Not breastfeeding increases rates of disease and the associated costs of treating disease and therefore increases the burden on community and hospital healthcare facilities (Rollins et al, 2016). One of the global Sustainable Development Goals is to reduce poverty and improve prosperity. Scaling up breastfeeding reduces inequality and disease burden and also provides optimal health. Thus, it is an obvious public health intervention that would have far-reaching positive economic impact, as well as clear benefits for individuals (Hansen, 2016).

If we think about why infants need milk, we often assume that human milk is primarily about nutrition. However, some evolutionary studies have found that the primary purpose of milk was for immunologic support, as well as optimising gut health (Bode, 2012). This makes sense of some of the components found in milk – such as indigestible human milk oligosaccharides or HMOs, whose primary function is to feed the prebiotics in the gut (Bode, 2015). Some of these prebiotics, such as *Bifidobacterium infantis*, serve to protect the infant from respiratory and gastrointestinal infections. Amazingly, these HMOs compete with the gut epithelial surface for the attachment of pathogens like rotavirus, norovirus, E. coli and campylobacter. The HMOs attach to these harmful pathogens which are then excreted harmlessly in stool rather than causing disease. The HMOs have absolutely no nutritional value whatsoever – they seem to be purely about immunological protection.

The human infant gut is not sterile at birth, as previously thought. However, the gut is far from completely 'seeded' with beneficial bacteria either. The infant immune system is incomplete, and many people acknowledge that human milk is designed to effectively 'complete' the immune system. Human milk contains active immunity in the form of immunoglobulins, also known as antibodies. In particular, Secretory Immunoglobulin A (SIgA) coats the lining of the gut, protecting it from the invasion of harmful pathogens, and is present in a dose-response amount in human milk for the first four months of life, and continues to be produced in smaller quantities for as long as milk is made. SIgA transfers across the placenta during pregnancy and is hugely valuable immunologically to newborns but infants cannot synthesise their own in the first few months after birth. Therefore, they are entirely dependent on receiving this via human milk (Bernt and Walker, 2001).

All mammals make species-specific milk for their young, and as uncomfortable as this truth is, feeding babies with non-species-specific milk in the form of infant formula, whilst it is nutritionally complete, does not provide optimal immunity. Thus, formula fed infants have a higher risk of many atopic, infectious, autoimmune and some malignancies, as well as SIDS, obesity, dental caries and malocclusion (Victora et al, 2016).

There is extraordinarily little research into this, but many mothers have told me that their sick child can digest breast milk when they cannot tolerate anything else, or that the continuation of breastfeeding has enabled them to have fewer nasogastric tube feeds. One mother I spoke to specifically felt that giving breast milk was worth the effort because her child was already working so hard to survive that she did not want to increase their burden of digestion by giving formula. She felt that breast milk was more efficient and caused her baby less discomfort and straining. This makes sense physiologically as the micro and macronutrients in human milk are more bioavailable and stools are often softer and easier to pass.

The language of 'prevention'

Much of the language around breastfeeding has historically discussed the 'benefits' of breastfeeding, and the 'reduction in risk' of disease if a child is breastfed. It is arguably more helpful for parents of sick children, as well as lactation advocates to acknowledge that breastfeeding confers a *normal* rate of *acquired* diseases and conditions in both lactating mothers and infants and children. There are other factors that affect our susceptibility to disease and infection, such as genetics, family history, environmental exposures, lifestyle, toxins and good old chance. It's not just about one factor, and it would be a mistake to think of human milk as being a panacea for all illnesses. Despite optimal infant and young child feeding, some breastfed infants or children do still develop illnesses that are seen at higher rates in their formula fed peers. The fact that breastfed children are less likely than formula fed children to become sick clearly does not render breast milk a guarantee for a disease-free childhood, and it also does not mean that feeding formula always causes harm. What it means for us is that the needs and challenges of breastfed infants and children who become unwell, as well as those with anatomical anomalies, accidents and trauma, disability and congenital conditions are important considerations that have not been adequately addressed in the literature.

As Stuebe (2009) points out, the language of breastfeeding *preventing* negative health outcomes or conferring *benefits* inadvertently presents formula feeding as the baseline, and breastfeeding as some kind of added bonus. Although formula is an essential and sometimes lifesaving part of infant feeding, it is not the biologically standard way to feed human infants. Therefore it is more accurate (though undoubtedly more emotive) to acknowledge that there are increased risks associated with formula feeding and reduced breastfeeding exclusivity and duration. I am well aware that while this may be true, it is also hard to hear, and it is never my intention to appear judgmental. It can be hard to read these kinds of public health messages without linking it to our personal stories. However, this message is aimed not at individuals but rather at system-wide approaches within healthcare settings that should be in place to protect breastfeeding and treat it as the norm. Perhaps we have not found the perfect way to describe this yet, but certainly many of the families that I support are very hurt by the idea that breastfeeding *should* have prevented illness, and yet didn't. There is no easy answer to language sometimes.

More accurate and nuanced use of language is particularly important when considering medically complex children. Of course breastfeeding is not just about immunological protection and nutritional content, but all the other positive aspects of the breastfeeding relationship which we shall return to later. Focusing on the language of prevention for just a while longer, describing breastfeeding as an intervention to reduce the risk of disease or certain conditions could arguably present a few problems in understanding:

1. That if children become sick, breastfeeding could be perceived to have 'failed' to work, to offer the protection that we expected. Clearly, we have no fortune telling abilities to be able to definitively say whether their disease or illness would have been worse without breastfeeding.

2. Breastfeeding has no role in preventing congenital conditions, disabilities, anatomical anomalies, or accidents and trauma. Therefore, this can feel irrelevant to children who present with these conditions.

3. If breastfeeding is seen as a public health intervention which prevents disease, the focus will be on prevention of illness instead of supporting parents to continue through medical challenges, with all the associated non-nutritional benefits of comfort and connection also being overlooked.

4. Not all illnesses and diseases have the same risk reduction with breastfeeding. For example, some conditions are only less prevalent when breastfeeding is exclusive, or with certain durations of breastfeeding (Victora et al, 2016). Therefore, it is not true to say that breastfeeding prevents all illnesses in the same way. For example, breastfeeding provides a dose-response effect to the risk of developing pneumonia, with more risk observed in less exclusively breastfed infants (Lamberti et al, 2013) and a systematic review found that breastfeeding reduces the risk of acute lymphoblastic leukaemia by 14-20% when children are breastfed for six months or more (Amitay and Keinan-Boker, 2015).

5. Some mothers who find breastfeeding difficult or expressing unmanageable (sometimes because of their child's medical challenges) may feel the added burden of guilt if they are unable to meet their breastfeeding goals.

6. This mindset also arguably positions breastfeeding as a medical intervention which can be quantified and analysed rather than a developmentally, relationally and socially normal part of mothering and parenting.

This is important on a human level, because sometimes parents have heard or been taught that breastfeeding 'reduces the risk' of those negative health outcomes. This may be upsetting or confusing for families of sick children, as they are sometimes optimally fed, and yet still have a serious illness. Some parents have felt 'short-changed', that they did something wrong, or that perhaps their milk wasn't special *enough*. The reason for this is that breastfeeding is associated with lower rates of illness, but does not guarantee immunity from these illnesses and conditions (Binns and Lee, 2019).

This may not be a widely held view, but I believe that if we make prevention of disease the focus of breastfeeding as a public health intervention, we fail to meet the needs of families whose children were breastfed, and yet became sick. For these families, the distinction between a normal level of risk, and an increased level of risk is important, to prevent them from feeling like breastfeeding has let them down. As the mother of a breastfed child who developed leukaemia, I don't feel like breastfeeding 'failed' to protect my child. However, I do see the need for more people to understand the difference between correlation and causation. The nuances of risk reduction are subtle, but it is important to ensure accurate and sensitive information is conveyed.

Human milk composition

Of course, human milk is also important for nutrition and growth. What is interesting about it is that the exact composition of milk varies by the infant's age, gestational stage, metabolic rate, gender, and presence of illness. It also fluctuates according to the time of day, and from day to day (Wambach and Spencer, 2021). The proportion of whey to casein shifts markedly in the first few weeks, from a 90:10 ratio in the early days and weeks, to 60:40 in mature milk. This shift in protein ratio is why breastfed infants' stooling patterns shift from the regular two to four stools per day to the less frequent pattern common among infants over 6 weeks (den Hertog et al, 2012).

The composition of milk adjusts to meet the changing needs of the infant or child, but broadly contains carbohydrate in the form of lactose, fats, and proteins, with immune factors, lactoferrin, lymphocytes and phagocytes, long chain polyunsaturated fatty acids like docosahexaenoic acid (DHA), lysozyme, cytokines, vitamins, minerals and many hormones. Human milk also mirrors the levels of the circadian hormones, cortisol and melatonin – with higher levels of melatonin in the evening according to the maternal circadian rhythm (Hahn-Holbrook et al, 2019).

Human milk contains stem cells at a rate of several thousand to millions of cells per feed, capable of differentiating into specialised cells and seeding infant organs. Human milk contains billions of cells, and when both the mother and child are healthy, the proportion of leukocytes (white blood cells) is less than 2% of this number. However, breastfeeding is a dynamic process and one of the mechanisms by which it is responsive is the retrograde inoculation theory – commonly known as 'backwash'. Infant saliva causes microbial cross talk with the mammary microbiome, effectively causing the milk to be altered in response to the infant's environmental exposure. Immunological crosstalk is via the gut-associated lymphoid tissue (GALT) and bronchus-associated lymphoid tissue (BALT) pathways which cause mammary tissue to produce specific SIgA antibodies (Goldman et al,

1983). The 'backwash' theory was first discussed by Hinde and Lewis (2015) and supported by evidence discovered by the CHILD study team (Moossavi et al, 2019). It was later expanded (Beghetti et al, 2019) though it remains a hypothesis. Essentially, during suckling, the theory suggests that a child's saliva enters the mammary tissue and via the entero-mammary pathway, affects the microbiota of the milk produced, meaning that the milk can be compositionally changed in response to infant exposure to pathogens.

The relevance to childhood illness is obvious - when either the mother or infant are unwell, white blood cells are recruited from the maternal bloodstream and make up a vastly increased proportion of these billions of cells in milk, evidencing the ability of the human breast to dynamically alter the composition of milk to adapt to the acute needs of the child for immunologic protection (Hassiotou and Hartmann, 2014). At times of acute infant infection, human milk has specifically been found to contain more leukocytes, macrophages, and tumour necrosis factor-α (TNFα), with these components returning to lower levels in the recovery phase (Riskin et al, 2012). SIgA specific antibodies are also present in human milk during times of acute infection, and these appear to remain for several months after the illness (Juncker et al, 2021). Like HMOs, SIgA is virtually unabsorbed, and its primary function is immunologic support, making sense of the increased concentrations found during acute illness.

Human milk is not always white, and can be coloured bright yellow in the beginning - colostrum is golden coloured due to the high levels of immunoglobulins. Many mothers notice that their milk changes colour when they or their babies are acutely unwell as the levels of immunoglobulins increase (Feist et al, 2000). Milk can also be coloured blue, green and pink due to highly pigmented foods such as beetroot or may look watery. Milk expressed in the morning is usually more plentiful in terms of volume, but proportionally lower in fat, whereas milk expressed at the end of the day is often lower in volume but higher in fat. These changes and fluctuations are normal, and although some parents worry about the quality or fat content of breast milk, it is rarely a problem. Never judge the quality of milk by its appearance – if the baby is growing well – the colour is irrelevant. Don't forget, if mothers were not expressing, we wouldn't even know.

The importance of breastfeeding for mothers

Breastfeeding is indisputably significant for infants and children, but it is also protective for the mother. Not breastfeeding is associated with higher rates of invasive breast cancer, ovarian cancer, diabetes, heart disease and being overweight (Victora et al, 2016). Among women who intend to breastfeed, rates of postnatal depression are lower when they meet their own self-defined breastfeeding goals. Rates of depression in the first six weeks are lower the longer and more exclusively they feed their children (Borra et al, 2015).

Breastfeeding causes oxytocin and prolactin to be released which improves maternal mood (Moore et al, 2016) and facilitates sleep (Avidan, 2007; Astbury et al, 2022). This response continues for as long as the child is held in skin to skin contact or breastfed, and thus is a mediating factor in postnatal mood (Kendall-Tackett, 2015), as well as eliciting a calming effect on mothers and children. Breastfeeding reduces blood pressure and cortisol levels and has long term impacts on cardiovascular health, reducing their risk of heart disease and stroke (Stuebe, 2015). A recent study has also suggested that breastfeeding may improve cognitive functioning in postmenopausal women. The study found that women who had breastfed performed better on tests of their memory, learning, executive functioning and processing speed. One possible hypothesis is that breastfeeding leads to improved stress regulation and the results suggest that breastfeeding protects against cognitive decline in later life (Fox et al, 2021).

It is thus valid and relevant that professionals invested in public health consider not only the impact of reduced breastfeeding duration and exclusivity on infants and children, but also on their mothers.

The importance of breastfeeding for sick children

Considering the importance in general of human milk as the norm for the human species, it is perhaps obvious that this is no less true for sick children. There are a number of properties and aspects of breastfeeding and human milk that are particularly relevant for this population. Fascinatingly, as well as immunological protection, human milk also contains endorphins and beta casein. These factors provide effective pain relief, and breastfeeding has been found to provide good pain relief during procedures such as routine immunisation (Shah et al, 2015; Harrison et al, 2016). Breastfeeding has not been evaluated for pain relieving efficacy with other procedures, such as blood tests and cannulation, but anecdotally it appears to provide excellent post painful-procedure comfort.

A parent's motivation for breastfeeding a sick child is individual, and this may vary from a pragmatic decision to continue doing what was previously working well for some, to an increased desire to provide immunologic factors to buffer them from additional disease burden or iatrogenic infection (Matthews et al, 1998; Brown and Shenker, 2022). Many of the parents I speak to tell me that their primary reason to breastfeed their children is for comfort, connection, and closeness. They describe breastfeeding being a link to normality, and providing a safe 'home' for their child at a time when everything else feels chaotic. Many parents also describe breastfeeding as a 'parenting tool' – a way to 'fix' upset, bored, frustrated, hurting and confused children.

Breastfeeding may also be a way for mothers to feel more integrally involved in their child's care, providing them with purpose and meaning. There is almost no research into this aspect within the paediatric setting, but borrowing literature from the neonatal intensive care setting can offer insight into the value that breastfeeding may have in terms of increased confidence, establishing an identity as a mother, involvement and sense of agency (Flacking et al, 2007; Butler et al, 2014; Mortensen et al, 2015). Emotional connection, comfort and stress-reduction through breastfeeding are also valid and important reasons to preserve it, and may be a way of connecting back to normality and home routines (Ekstrom and Nissen, 2006; Murray et al, 2007; Moberg and Prime, 2013).

As mentioned, breast milk contains numerous known and unknown immunologic components including secretory IgA, lymphocytes, macrophages, lysozyme and lactoferrin (Lawrence, 2022), and reduces exposure to foreign proteins (Järvinen et al, 2019). Breastfed infants with severe pneumonia in one study had fewer days of ventilation, less iatrogenic infection and fewer days in hospital (Laguna-Cruz and Becina, 2017). Other studies find that breastfed children have fewer complications and less severe illness overall (Quigley et al, 2009; Rodriguez et al, 2005).

While the importance of breastfeeding for maternal and child health is well understood in a general sense, and also for preterm infants, there is very little research exploring how and why it is harder to breastfeed medically complex infants and children beyond the neonatal period. This group of children may particularly benefit from the immunological components of human milk, and breastfeeding can be a physical and emotional comfort to both parents and children. Breastfeeding can continue to provide a substantial amount of calories, micro and macronutrients and immunological components into the second year of life and beyond (Dewey et al, 1984; Czosnykowska-Łukacka et al, 2018; Doherty et al, 2018; Lackey et al, 2021). We also know that among parents whose breastfeeding journey ends before they planned, many experience feelings of sadness and disappointment (Brown, 2018).

There are therefore numerous reasons that point to the need to protect and promote breastfeeding in the medically complex population. Optimising infant feeding is likely to also provide a greater sense of self-efficacy for mothers and families, and provides an obvious opportunity for family centred care (FCC) and parent involvement.

Chapter 2

How breastfeeding works

In order to understand how breastfeeding might be more difficult to achieve for a sick or medically complex child, we need to understand how it works in a general sense. There are many excellent books that exhaustively cover the mechanics of breastfeeding in far greater detail. I highly recommend *The Womanly Art of Breastfeeding* (La Leche League), *A Guide to Supporting Breastfeeding for the Medical Profession* (Brown and Jones, 2019) and *The Positive Breastfeeding Book* (Brown, 2018) as accessible books. This book provides only a brief overview, as its focus is on the medically complex population. We'll start by exploring how to facilitate optimal breastfeeding. I'm very aware of the range of lactation expertise as you approach this chapter. If you're already knowledgeable about breastfeeding then consider the next two chapters' revision, or skip ahead to chapter 4 to get straight to the specifics of sick children.

There are many known protective factors that enable parents to achieve their breastfeeding goals. Good preparation and antenatal education has been found to support breastfeeding self-efficacy. More breastfeeding knowledge has been found to be associated with longer and more exclusive breastfeeding rates (Zhang et al, 2018). Alongside knowledge of how breastfeeding works, and how to overcome common hurdles, realistic expectations of normal infant behaviour, frequency of feeding, and feeding responsively are also supportive (Brown and Arnott, 2014). Intention and motivation to breastfeed is a significant buffering factor. Mothers who believe that breastfeeding is important for their child were more likely to want to breastfeed exclusively, and the higher the level of motivation, the more likely they were to achieve this goal. Motivation has also been found to be predictive of a longer duration of breastfeeding (Martin et al, 2021).

Having a supportive partner is known to be an important factor in the establishment and maintenance of breastfeeding (Clifford and McIntyre, 2008), as well as the influence of the maternal grandmother. Higher rates of breastfeeding seen in families where the parents were themselves breastfed (Negin et al, 2016). Higher rates of breastfeeding exclusivity and duration are also seen when there is a positive culture of breastfeeding – whether this comes from peers, religious institutions, the community, wider family members, healthcare professionals, media influencers or the workplace (Chang et al, 2021). Community support is well-known to have a positive impact, and this support should be universally offered but individually tailored, ongoing, and ideally face-to-face (McFadden et al, 2016). Although support is often offered by professionals, lay or peer supporters have been shown to successfully augment services by providing friendly, accessible, positive interactions with breastfeeding mothers (Trickey et al, 2018).

Previous breastfeeding experience appears to have a mixed effect on breastfeeding duration and exclusivity. Studies have found that a previous positive experience of breastfeeding with a first child predicts longer breastfeeding duration with subsequent children (Sutherland et al, 2012). However, in general, unsuccessful attempts to breastfeed a first child, breastfeeding less exclusively or for a shorter duration is strongly predictive of shorter breastfeeding duration or non-initiation of breastfeeding with a subsequent child (Bai et al, 2015).

There are numerous demographic characteristics that have been studied in relation to their respective effects on breastfeeding duration and exclusivity. Mothers who are older than 30, have higher socioeconomic status, and higher educational level are most likely to breastfeed in the UK (Simpson et al, 2019; Sarki et al, 2019). Breastfeeding has been felt by some researchers to be a parenting practice of privilege, perhaps due to better access to antenatal education, more confidence, and more ability to overcome some of the societal barriers to breastfeeding (Smith, 2018).

Ethnicity also has an influence on breastfeeding rates, and in the UK, non-white mothers are more likely to breastfeed (Simpson et al, 2021), though second and third generation immigrants have been shown to increasingly adopt the local customs, causing a decline in culturally normal breastfeeding rates (Marvin-Dowle et al, 2021). This finding contrasts with other data from different countries that suggests that Black, Asian and Mixed-race parents are less likely than their white peers to meet their personal feeding goals due to complex issues of institutional racism, prejudice and inequality of access (Hamner et al, 2021).

There are many known protective factors surrounding the birth and immediate postpartum that can affect breastfeeding. Of course mothers will bring a complex and varied background of influencing factors as they begin to feed and care for their child. However, we must also acknowledge the impact of healthcare experiences, healthcare professional attitudes, staff interactions and the level of available support that parents experience in the hospital setting. Being born in a BFI accredited hospital has been found to increase the rates of initiation of breastfeeding and breastfeeding in the first week of life, though this has not been clearly shown to have a sustained impact. Training community health visitors in lactation support has been found to reduce breastfeeding cessation, as does adopting a hands-off approach to breastfeeding support (Fallon et al, 2019). Type of birth has also been shown to impact breastfeeding, with higher rates of breastfeeding seen among women who had a vaginal birth rather than a caesarean birth (Zhang et al, 2019; Chen et al, 2018). Early and prolonged skin-to-skin contact has long been known to facilitate breastfeeding, as well as optimise infant physiological adaptation to the stress of birth (Bergman et al, 2019). Skin-to-skin contact has no upper time limit, and an abundance of literature points to this intervention being appropriate for sick and low birth weight neonates, and those undergoing painful needlestick procedures, and may additionally enhance weight gain (Johnston et al, 2009; Blomqvist and Nyqvist, 2011; Salim et al, 2021; Charpak et al, 2021).

Frustratingly, there are no studies of skin-to-skin in the paediatric setting, so we only have studies exploring the impact in preterm neonates, and healthy newborns. However, logically, there is no physiological reason why skin-to-skin would not be just as beneficial for sick infants and children beyond the neonatal period, and we can look to the evidence that carrying infants and young children is considered by many to be the anthropological norm (Berecz et al, 2020) and some research points to the general positive effect of touch (Pawling et al, 2017).

Keeping mothers and infants together as much as possible is a key part of facilitating effective breastfeeding and optimising a mother's milk supply (WHO, 2018), with no separation unless absolutely necessary. Even when mothers are hospitalised, best practice is to allow the infant to remain with their mother (Bartick et al, 2021). Beyond the immediate postpartum period, discussions around proximity and infant sleep location remain important. It is known that mothers who sleep in close proximity to their infants are better able to respond promptly to early feeding cues, supporting more cue-based care which is protective of optimal feeding (Brown and Arnott, 2014; Ventura, 2017; Little et al, 2018). Bedsharing while breastfeeding, coined 'breastsleeping' (McKenna and Gettler, 2016) facilitates more rest and thus makes breastfeeding for longer durations more sustainable for parents (McKenna et al, 2007; ABM, 2008).

Bedsharing is a contentious issue even outside the hospital setting, but when we add in a small hospital bed, unforgiving hard floors, compromised infants with evolving or unknown conditions, risk factors and vulnerabilities, it becomes a minefield. Yet, if we prohibit bed sharing in hospitals, and insist that children remain in hospital cots, this can lead to unsettled infants, sleepless nights for parents and distress. Inevitably, some parents end up holding their infants upright against their bodies all night, or bringing them into the parent pull-out bed or chair – both environments that are arguably much riskier, and yet there probably isn't an easy answer.

Considering how all these protective factors apply to the sick child in hospital, it is clear that some are difficult to achieve when a sick or medically complex child is admitted to hospital. While some protective interventions may be possible to maintain, several are hindered by the staff, logistics, culture or environment of the paediatric ward - particularly in relation to paediatric healthcare professional training, proximity measures, peer support and community interventions.

How breast milk is made

Having considered the general practices and interventions that make breastfeeding possible, let's move on to think about the specifics, beginning with milk supply.

The human breast starts developing functional glandular tissue during puberty and continues throughout adolescence and early adulthood. However, it only completes its development during pregnancy. Under the influence of progesterone, oestrogen, prolactin, human placental lactogen and growth hormone, glandular milk producing tissue develops and milk begins to be produced in the alveoli (milk making cells) during the early part of the second trimester.

Most pregnant mothers notice breast and nipple changes, such as tingling, fullness, aching, and changing shape and colour of their breasts, nipples and areolas. They may notice prominent veins appearing in their breasts, as well as sometimes some leaking of milk. While increases in breast size and the appearance of visible veins are a positive sign that the breast is undergoing important development in readiness for lactation, the presence or absence of leaking in pregnancy is not a reliable indicator of potential milk supply.

Breast development accelerates rapidly in the second half of the pregnancy, but copious milk production is inhibited by high levels of progesterone which block the action of prolactin within the alveolar cells.

Copious milk production, (known as lactogenesis II) is triggered by the drop in progesterone caused by the birth of the placenta. There is a slight delay of between two to five days before milk begins to be produced in larger quantities, and until this time, infants access nutrient-dense but small volumes of colostrum. After the onset of lactogenesis II, milk volumes gradually increase.

Initially, most mothers' milk producing *capacity* far exceeds infant need – there are many more alveolar cells in most breasts than are required for one infant. Ongoing milk production, and the regulation of milk supply is driven by milk removal. The rate of milk synthesis is related to the degree of breast fullness, so fuller breasts make milk more slowly than more well drained breasts. This is a brilliant and efficient mechanism to ensure that valuable energy is not wasted on milk production if it is not required (and why we don't explode!). Therefore, the best way to keep the rate of milk synthesis high is frequent, effective milk removal. Conversely, the best way to reduce milk supply is to stretch out the time between feeds or expressing sessions, allowing milk to build up in the breast. This is one reason why trying to get babies to feed on an infrequent feeding routine, such as every three to four hours is so detrimental to the milk supply. Breastfeeding works best when it is done responsively.

The amount of milk an individual breast can hold is variable, both between breasts and between mothers. Many mothers report having one breast that produces a significant amount more milk than the other side – which is one reason not to assign sides to multiples for instance. Some studies have reported women being able to store up to 600ml of milk per breast, versus others whose milk storage capacity may be less than 100ml (Daly et al, 1993). The milk storage capacity affects how frequently infants need to feed but does not affect the ability to produce a full milk supply. This means that a breast with smaller storage capacity can still perfectly adequately feed a baby, but the baby may need to feed more frequently in order to access every drop of the available milk. (By the way, this has nothing to do with the visible size of the breast - appearances can be deceiving!)

I often use an analogy of an electric car. Some electric vehicles can drive for over 300 miles before they need to be charged, whereas others only have a 30-50 mile range. If you assume you're 'driving' a long-range car and feed infrequently, when you actually have a short-range car, you'll run into problems. If you'll bear with the car analogy a little longer, you will basically 'run out of fuel'. The frustrating thing about this is that a 'breastfeeding breakdown' of this type is unrelated to milk making potential, and wholly attributable to breastfeeding mismanagement or misunderstanding.

A breast with a large storage capacity may mean that an infant can feed infrequently, and the milk supply may not be affected. Of course, this also relies on the infant being able to drink a large volume in one feed, which is not guaranteed because everyone, even an infant, has varying appetites and stomach capacities. These are some of the many reasons why responsive feeding is recommended. If we do not know the storage capacity of the mother, or the stomach capacity of the infant, it is safest to recommend that infants are simply allowed to cue their feeding, and mothers are encouraged to feed their infants as often as they show these feeding cues. We will come back later to when we need to intervene - if for example infants *do not* cue to feed.

Supporting effective early feeding

There are plenty of practical ways to both passively and actively support effective early feeding. Primarily, it is important to remember that for the infant, finessing feeding can take some practice, healthy term infants have all the reflexes they need to get to the breast, initiate suckling and regulate their milk intake. Therefore, facilitating immediate skin-to-skin and encouraging early, infant-led self-attachment with a hands-off approach and very little interference is ideal, if possible, since the early feeds imprint suckling behaviours. Touching infants on the back of their head while they are trying to feed, swaddling them, holding their hands or pushing them on to the breast can make them confused and distressed. Disturbing infants, forcing them to feed, or getting in the way of those reflexes can disturb rooting and tongue placement. It is also advisable to discourage suckling on pacifiers and bottle teats for the same reason until breastfeeding is established. While some infants seem to be able to transition between the breast and a teat with no apparent difficulty, others struggle, particularly if breastfeeding has not yet been established. Only give additional fluids or formula if medically indicated, and finally, encourage parents to get early skilled support if they need it.

More specific ways to optimise feeding include suggestions for how to best facilitate the innate behaviours of the newborn. Infants expect to feed in a prone position, and use their chests, arms, knees, feet and most of their face to locate the breast and attach successfully. Many infants will panic when held in a classic cradle hold, because their feet are unsupported, and gravity is pulling them down and away from the breast, meaning that they can't use their rooting, stepping and crawling reflexes to find the breast (Milinco et al, 2020). There is a greater tendency to see more disorganised behaviours when infants are held so that they are lying on their backs looking up at the breast, leading with their chin (Douglas and Keogh, 2017).

I often explain that infants who are positioned on their backs behave in a very similar way to a beetle on their back. A beetle the wrong way up tends to wave its legs around in a disorganised fashion and can't get to where they want to be. Place them the right way round and they know exactly what to do. Babies are kind of the same. Keep them in a gravity friendly position (Colson et al, 2008), and keep their face in constant contact with the breast so that they can use their cheeks, mouth, chin and jaw to attach properly. Adult hands need to be away from the back of the infant's head and cheeks so as not to confuse these innate behaviours. You will also probably find that infants prefer to have their head higher than their hips, so that they are lying either obliquely across their parent's abdomen or held upright.

Normal feed volumes

As soon as infants are born, they are able to access colostrum, which is thick and sticky (like nectar) and very low in volume, although very nutrient dense. The average newborn has been found to consume about 37ml in the first 24 hours, or approximately 7ml per feed – only a little more than a teaspoon. One study found that the first 24-hour fluid intake was closer to 22ml (Hester et al, 2012). This is not to suggest that these normal volumes should be measured or aimed for outside of a research setting, but they provide useful validation of the normalcy of these low volumes in the early days. These small volumes increase gradually over the first one to three days, and then much more rapidly from about day four or five. The onset of copious milk production is called lactogenesis II and as you may remember, it is triggered by the delivery of the placenta and consequent drop in progesterone.

By 7-14 days, a healthy-term singleton baby drinks between 550-1150ml of milk in 24 hours (Cox et al, 1996). I appreciate that this is a large variation, which is explained by differences in infant size, metabolic rate and other factors (Ramsay et al, 2005). The amount of milk an infant consumes does not significantly increase between one to six months and averages about 800ml in 24 hours (Daly et al, 1993; Kent et al, 2013). While an infant's growth and nutrient needs change, the fluctuations in milk composition accommodate these changes in nutritional needs, without the need for a significant increase in volume. This is important to know, especially within paediatrics, as formula-fed babies will need more milk the bigger and older they get, and many healthcare professionals assume that breast milk volumes similarly increase with a child's age and weight. In fact, many from a clinical paediatric background will be familiar with fluid volume calculations based on infant weight. These calculations are inappropriate for healthy, thriving breastfed infants, and even among formula-fed infants, there is a concern that some infants are being overfed.

With an established milk supply, most infants only access about two thirds of the available milk volume, so the breast is never 'empty' (Wambach and Spencer, 2021). Infants themselves regulate their milk intake through appetite regulation hormones including cholecystokinin, ghrelin, leptin and brain derived neurotrophic factor which increase feelings of satiety, trigger spontaneous release of the breast, and promote deep sleep (Cordeira and Rios, 2011; Shukla and Basheer, 2016; Larson-Meyer et al, 2021). This is one reason it is so hard to try to get infants into a 'feed-play-sleep' routine – they are naturally wired to fall asleep while feeding.

Interestingly, in one study, second time mothers produced significantly more milk by their child's second week, though the volumes evened out by four weeks, so if parents had a hard time breastfeeding their first child, they may be reassured to know that it may be very different second or third time around (Ingram et al, 2001).

Normal infant growth

You will be aware that almost all infants lose weight as part of the physiological fluid loss after birth. This initial weight loss is more marked among babies born by caesarean section and those whose mothers received IV fluids in labour. The nadir in weight tends to occur around day 3, usually right before the onset of copious milk production, and from that point they should begin to gain weight. The tolerance for weight loss is contested, with upper limits around 7% reported in the literature (Noel-Weiss et al, 2008) and one study found that higher levels of weight loss are correlated with more significant jaundice - though this was unrelated to breastfeeding per se (Yang et al, 2013).

Recent weight loss nomograms based on a large cohort of term neonates have helped to identify those infants at greater risk of weight loss earlier, and have found that on average, newborns lose between 5-10% of their birth weight depending on the mode of birth

(Flaherman et al, 2015). With fully optimised feeding, the weight loss can be even lower and keeping parents and babies in uninterrupted skin to skin and promoting very frequent effective feeding seems to be an important intervention (Flaherman et al, 2017).

If newborns lose 8-10% of their birth weight this should trigger a prompt feeding assessment and additional support to optimise feeding efficiency. More than 10% weight loss is associated with higher rates of hospital admission although routine supplementation with formula is not *necessarily* clinically required if good feeding support can be accessed and the infant can be safely and closely monitored. Indeed, some studies find an association of lower percentage weight loss with earlier and more effective breastfeeding support.

According to studies, 75% of newborns regain their birth weight by seven days post birth, with more than 97% regaining birth weight by 21 days (Grossman et al, 2012). If feeding and weight challenges are encountered, prompt skilled feeding support is essential so changes can be made which will optimise the feeding outcome before it escalates.

How to identify effective feeding

Being able to identify effective feeding is essential for anyone working with infants and mothers. It's not just a matter of confirming that an infant is on the breast and doing *something*. In other words, just because the baby is on the breast and moving their mouth a bit, does not necessarily mean that they are effectively feeding.

The behaviour of the infant changes throughout a feed. When an infant starts to suckle, the oxytocin response in the mother triggers the spontaneous milk ejection reflex. This causes a ring of muscle cells around each milk-making cell to contract, and milk is squeezed out into the milk ducts. Thus, with the milk ejection reflex (colloquially known as the let-down reflex) milk will start to drip or spray. The infant may passively swallow this milk as it sprays into their mouth. Some mothers experience a discernible tingling, aching or cramping sensation in their breast as this happens. However, whether or not a mother feels the let-down is not a good indication that it has occurred.

The mother will have several milk ejections per feed, with one study (Kent et al, 2008) finding that the average number of milk ejections was four (range 1-12). The amount of milk per milk ejection is related to the degree of breast fullness, and the volume of milk delivered during the milk ejection reflex is reduced with each milk ejection. In the study, after four milk ejections, babies received 99% of the available milk (which of course does not mean that the breast is empty).

Once this let-down has finished, the infant controls milk intake with their suckling behaviour, and the fat content gradually increases through the length of the feed, until the infant has had enough and spontaneously releases the breast. This fluctuation in flow rate and fat content affects the suckling behaviour of the infant. We must be able to identify that the infant is well attached, displaying a rhythmic, organised suck-swallow pattern and audible swallows that sound like little sighs are heard. While at the start of a feed you may hear a gulping noise, the swallowing quickly shifts to a quieter sound (it sounds like 'hup-ah' or is sometimes described as sounding like a sigh) and ends with infrequent swallows and flutter sucking. Many parents have found it helpful to understand how to observe effective feeding by listening to these noises and watch their infant's jaw working. As the jaw drops and pauses, the infant is usually heard swallowing. Once a parent is able to recognize this for themselves as effective feeding, they will know when to be concerned that their infant is not feeding efficiently. There are other softer and more subtle signs that milk is being transferred as well – such as the overall body posture of the infant. You will probably notice that their face looks relaxed and their hands are unclenched.

An experienced lactation professional will be able to spot an infant who is feeding ineffectively at the breast very quickly. If the attachment is not optimised, it can be very difficult for an infant to effectively feed. They sometimes suckle a little at the breast and exhibit a behaviour I call 'let-down surfing'. Essentially, the mother will experience a let-down reflex, which the infant will passively swallow and drink, but once the let-down is over, the infant may go back to soft suckling with no/few swallows. Since the mother may experience several let downs in the course of the feed, the infant may simply suckle until there is another let-down. This may, to the untrained eye, look like an effective feed, but in reality, the infant is not drinking effectively and efficiently. Feeds are likely to be long, frequent and often painful. Of course, how the infant responds to this depends on multiple factors, including their temperament, how sleepy they are and more. Some infants will fuss and cry, be restless and unhappy all the time unless they are being fed, while others will simply suckle quietly without pulling off. This is why it is so important to assess the feed quality, and also monitor objective criteria - nappies and weight.

Effective feeding should also be pain (though not sensation) free. It is normal for mothers to experience a very strong pulling sensation, and in the early days, it may also feel tender and a little uncomfortable for some. Being able to identify whether pain is hormonal, or mechanical is very important. I find it helps to remind mothers that when they first became pregnant, their nipples were also tender and sensitive – it is related to hormonal sensitivity, as well as getting used to breastfeeding. Common wisdom is that if feeding is uncomfortable, requiring concentration and slow breathing for up to 10-20 seconds, this is normal. If the mother is curling her toes, scrunching her eyes shut, unable to speak, or cursing, the chances are the positioning and attachment aren't great.

After the initial weight loss, we should see a weight gain of between 20-30g per day in healthy infants with no underlying conditions, depending on the age of the child and their gender, with boys gaining slightly more per day than girls, but growth should always be plotted on the centile chart to see weight gain in context. The growth rate does slow at around four months from around 200g per week to 115g per week. Finally, it's important to be aware of normal voiding patterns. Often, infants will continue to produce wet nappies even if their weight is faltering. Stools are a better indicator of satisfactory weight gain and optimal feeding. Breastfed infants tend to stool more frequently than formula fed infants, and indeed, a systematic review and meta-analysis found that breastfed infants are significantly less likely to be constipated at 3 months (Koppen et al, 2018). Some studies suggest up to four stools per day (den Hertog et al, 2012), while the Baby Friendly Initiative (BFI) in the UK suggests two stools as a minimum until about four to six weeks. Any infant who is not voiding and stooling adequately should have their feeding evaluated by someone skilled in assessing feeding, with appropriate support and intervention put in place to optimise infant growth, health and nutrition.

Normal infant feeding behaviour

As well as evaluating whether an infant is feeding effectively and assessing their weight, it is helpful for professionals to understand normal infant feeding behaviour, as this can differ from societal expectations, and even previous, more dated training. Infants rarely spontaneously feed according to a robust predictable schedule, but tend to feed frequently, with some bursts of more frequent feeding. Trying to push infants into a strict schedule will only work for a small proportion of infants, and evidence suggests that if the baby does not fall into this pattern easily, the level of stress and rates of depression in parents is higher. In addition, there are more likely to be breastfeeding problems and higher rates of breastfeeding cessation (Harries and Brown, 2017).

The number of feeds in 24 hours varies in the literature from 8 to 16 feeds, and the feed length is also variable, both between infants, and from feed to feed. The average length of feed is 5-40 minutes, and infants should finish the first breast first, before being offered the second. Some infants always want to drink from both breasts, while others never do.

The quality and efficiency of the feed is more significant than how many minutes. Often, parents and professionals may be tempted to try to quantify feeding efficiency and milk transfer by timing the length of the feed. This is not an accurate way to measure feeding.

Writing down 8, 11 or 20 minutes on an oral feed chart means nothing if the baby merely had a nap at the breast, and similarly, writing down five minutes on the chart does not mean that the infant only ingested a very small volume if they were gulping and guzzling efficiently. How long a feed lasts depends a little on the milk flow rate, a little on the infant's feeding style and mood, and a lot on how well the infant is positioned at the breast. Equating long feeds with large volumes, and short feeds with small volumes is an inherently flawed way to measure intake.

There are also some other normal behaviours that are often misunderstood. For example, feeding at night is normal and common, and in large studies, 70% of infants aged 6-18 months woke one to three times in the night for a feed (Hysing et al, 2014). It is normal to feed to sleep, and also to have periods of cluster feeding (where infants may feed on and off for a few hours), especially in the evening. Milk volumes are naturally lower in the evening, but this is not because the mother has 'run out of milk' or due to maternal fatigue, but a natural diurnal variation in milk volumes. The lower volumes are also associated with a higher fat content, and milk will mirror the blood circadian hormone profile of the mother – so melatonin levels in milk are higher in the evening. We don't need to overthink this. I have heard some parents worrying that giving their baby milk which was expressed in the morning is akin to giving their child a baby espresso. While it is true that milk mirrors the hormone levels present in blood, these variations are unlikely to make a drastic difference to infant alertness in the grand scheme of things. The bottom line is that all breast milk is good milk. If all you have to feed a baby at 11pm is milk pumped at 9am - go ahead and use it.

Frequent feeding, or cluster feeding in the evening does not necessarily indicate a low milk supply, even if a baby will take a bottle of the offered supplement. A common suggestion to establish whether an infant is cluster feeding due to hunger is to offer a baby a bottle of formula. This is rarely necessary and can lead to what is known colloquially as the 'top up trap'. Essentially, the more you top a baby up with formula, the less they will feed from the breast, and the breast will become fuller, signalling a downregulation of milk. Thus, a common scenario is the perception of low milk supply based on misinterpreting normal infant behaviour, then the action taken to address this normal infant behaviour leads to an actual low milk supply (Hookway, 2016). It's a self-fulfilling prophecy.

A better way to work out whether an infant is getting enough milk is to reassure and educate parents about counting nappies/diapers, and monitoring weight as frequently as recommended by their health care professional.

Parental self-doubt around milk supply is particularly common around six weeks – I call it the six-week triple whammy, because three changes often take place at the same time:

1. Milk production settles down, and it's common for mothers to report that their breasts feel softer, are less prone to leaking, and there is less perceptible difference between breast firmness before and after a feed.

2. The infant's rate of stooling often slows around this point, from at least two to four stools per day, to sometimes just a handful of stools per week (and sometimes less). Having successfully impressed upon parents the importance of counting nappies, they are sometimes concerned by this drop-off in stool production.

3. Infants are undergoing a huge number of developmental changes at around six weeks, and are commonly fussy, requiring more comfort and feeding, and often sleeping more erratically.

The triple whammy can really dent parental confidence if they don't know to expect it. It's a very common time for parents to start topping up with formula, often alongside a mother or parent describing that breastfeeding was going well, and then they 'couldn't keep up' with their baby's increased needs. The perception of low milk supply driven by fussier infant behaviour and increased need to comfort feed is particularly sad since we know that the milk volume does not significantly increase between one to six months, so by six weeks, milk volumes are already at their maximum. I know this can sound implausible, but it is because the composition of human milk varies constantly to meet the changing needs of the child via complex metabolic programming that starts in utero and seems to be mostly determined by infant feeding behaviour in the first month of life. About half the calories in milk are in the fat, and milk of older infants and toddlers contains more fat, which enables them to grow optimally despite not vastly increasing milk volume (Daly et al, 1993; Ramsay et al, 2005; Mandel et al, 2005; Kent et al, 2013).

This is one reason why I'm not a huge fan of describing these periods of infant fussing and developmental phases as 'growth spurts'. This implies that because an infant is growing, they will need substantially more milk. Parents often interpret this increased feeding as an infant trying to 'boost' milk supply and may become anxious that there isn't enough. More frequent feeding certainly does help to regulate and increase milk production in the early days, but not once milk volumes reach their maximum level.

It's therefore important to educate parents about:

- The stability of milk volumes between one and six months.
- The normality of infant behaviour and feeding patterns around developmental phases, especially at six weeks.
- The importance of viewing feeding as more than nutrition, but as a parenting tool and a valid source of comfort.

The truth is that infants feed more frequently for many reasons, including for comfort. They may access lower volume but more fatty milk during these periods of frequent feeding and more fully drain the breast which might be why some women feel like they are 'empty'. They are not empty - they may just be more well-drained than usual. Finally, it is normal for infants to have a fussy period after some feeds at any age – again, this does not indicate low milk supply in the absence of concrete signs of low milk intake. Babies, like all of us, are sometimes tired, bored, cranky, distracted, frustrated, overwhelmed or having a bad day. Supporting parents to be *curious* about their infant's behaviour and cues will help boost attunement and reciprocity, and also reduce self-doubt.

Growth charts

If you have concerns about a child's growth, you should look at their centile chart and review it in the context of their previous recorded weights. The World Health Organisation growth charts have now been adopted for all children, and these are based on global data from breastfed children as the baseline since previous charts were based on formula fed infants we now know to have been overfed. The Royal College of Paediatrics and Child Health has some great resources on growth and centile charts that you can access, and you can also download other appropriate growth charts – for example the chart for children with Trisomy 21, or children who were very preterm or have significant early health problems should be plotted on the neonatal and infant close monitoring chart. When caring for a child who may have growth concerns, the paediatric health professionals reading this will know that a detailed history is needed, along with ruling out organic and underlying causes, including, sadly, neglect and abuse (NICE, 2018).

Faltering growth is the term used to describe a child whose growth is not as expected. They may be gaining weight at a slower rate than would be considered optimal for them, not gaining weight at all, or losing weight. The term has replaced the older and much more punitive and emotive term 'failure to thrive' which can make many parents feel blamed. The NICE guideline classifies faltering growth as a child whose weight crosses two centiles if they were born between the 9th and the 91st centile, just one centile if their birth weight is under the 9th centile, and three centiles if their birth weight was above the 91st centile. In addition to the weight parameter, a child should be reviewed if their length or height is two centiles below the mid parental centile. These different thresholds of concern are based on several studies that aim to balance the need to accurately identify children who are at risk of under-nutrition, whilst also ensuring that the threshold is sensitive enough to only pick up those children at risk.

The Baby Friendly Standards/BFHI

You may be familiar with the Baby Friendly Standards as well as the Baby Friendly Hospital Initiative (BFHI), 'Ten Steps to Successful Breastfeeding'. The UK BFI is slightly different to the BFHI, in that it has a set of standards that apply to different clinical settings. However, there are many similarities. Both require a written breastfeeding policy that is communicated to all staff, and both share a requirement that health professionals who come into contact with parents and infants should be educated in the basic fundamentals of feeding support. In the UK, this also includes responsive parenting and paced bottle feeding.

UK Baby Friendly:

Stage 1: A Firm Foundation

Stage 2: An Educated Workforce

Stage 3: Parental experience in:

- Maternity Unit
- Neonatal Unit

- HV Services
- Children's Centres

Follow up Stage: Achieving sustainability.

In the UK, units who wish to undergo baby friendly accreditation must demonstrate commitment and provide a staff education program appropriate to the roles of the individuals. Finally, to ensure that these interventions are translated into demonstrable improvements in practice and positive care experiences, the experiences of parents as well as staff knowledge are audited annually. The standards are nuanced for different environments, but as yet, there is no provision for the paediatric setting, although plans are underway.

While sharing many similar priorities, the BFHI is slightly different:

1. Have a breastfeeding policy.
2. Educate health professionals who care for new parents and infants.
3. Educate parents and family members antenatally.
4. Support immediate initiation of breastfeeding.
5. Show mothers how to breastfeed and if separation is required, teach them how to maintain milk supply.
6. Give no other food or drink to babies unless medically indicated.
7. 'Rooming-in' 24 hours a day.
8. Encourage responsive/cue-based feeding.
9. Do not use pacifiers/ dummies or bottles.
10. Encourage support groups and provide resources at discharge from hospital.

The BFI has demonstrated positive impacts on the initiation of breastfeeding, though there is less evidence that it is significantly improving the duration of breastfeeding at this time (Perez-Escamilla et al, 2016), although this may be due to lack of consistency throughout services. However, my recent survey of healthcare professionals did find a statistically significant correlation between breastfeeding clinical skill scores and level of training. Indeed, *any* breastfeeding training was associated with greater confidence and skills, so while there are no paediatric-specific training programs at the time of writing, it is likely that *any* training is better than no training.

How babies feed

I'm now going to cover some of the specifics and mechanisms of feeding, and, as I do so, I want you to try to read this through the lens of considering the impact of these physiological functions if an infant is compromised.

Primarily, when an infant is positioned for breastfeeding, touching the middle lower lip stimulates the trigeminal nerve which triggers the infant to open wide in a gape. Then, as the infant moves towards the breast, the nipple, areola and some of the underlying breast tissue are drawn into the infant's mouth, with the tongue, lips and cheeks forming a seal to create a vacuum. The tongue tip remains over the lower gum ridge, while the lateral aspects of the tongue form a groove around the nipple and areola.

The nipple elongates and extends to near the junction of the hard and soft palate, triggering the infant suckle reflex. The lower jaw drops, which creates a pressure gradient and milk is pulled out of the breast. Tongue movements then organise the suckle and propel milk into the pharynx as the jaw closes. Just prior to the swallow, the airway closes to prevent aspiration, and once milk is in the oesophagus, the airway reopens.

The cycle can then start again. It's actually a remarkable operation (and is obviously a very different mechanism to bottle feeding), and infants need to coordinate sucking, swallowing and breathing, so it is normal for them to feed in bursts and pauses. Less gestationally mature infants tend to have shorter bursts of suckling, and more disorganised suckling patterns.

Infants are obligatory nose-breathers, though they may temporarily breathe through their mouths if they have some degree of compromise – such as a blocked nose. Their suckling reflex is present from about 28 weeks, and most papers suggest that it is mature by about 34 weeks gestational age, though there will always be people (including me) who know of babies far less gestationally mature than this who seem to get the hang of feeding earlier!

Physiological stress during breast/bottle feeding

It's important to note that oral feeding does present a physiological challenge to infants, even those who are healthy, with oxygen saturation levels falling to as low as 95% during a feed, and 92% after a feed (Hammerman and Kaplan, 1995). Coordinating suckling, swallowing and breathing requires numerous muscles, bones and cranial nerves to produce an organised sequence. One of the things that always blows my mind is that an average newborn respiratory rate is about 40-60 breaths per minute, or up to one breath per second. A swallow takes just over half a second. So every second, an infant potentially has to coordinate the sequence I have just described. It really is remarkable, even with an uncompromised infant. One study recorded and observed ten infants on ten separate occasions, over the first year of life to ascertain normative behaviours of respiration, swallowing and suckling, which amounted to an analysis of over 15,000 swallows. The researchers found that infants experience several maturational changes to their suck-swallow-breathe pattern in the first week of life, and then a further significant maturation to an adult-like breathing-swallowing pattern is observed at around six months of age (Kelly et al, 2007).

But if feeding creates a degree of normal physiological stress, are there differences between breast and bottle-fed infants? Well, yes. Multiple studies find that compared with bottle feeding, breastfed infants experience less oxygen desaturation, less bradycardias, less temperature fluctuation, more stable respirations and more coordinated swallow patterns (Chen et al, 2000; Goldfield et al, 2006; Moral et al, 2010). They also have their entire palate filled with breast tissue which optimises palate development and allows for optimal mandibular or jaw action. Breastfeeding also involves both nutritive as well as non-nutritive suckling, which is great for pain relief and comfort. A breastfed infant is also more able to control the flow of milk by adjusting their suckling rate.

This is important, because often in the clinical setting, breastfeeding is wrongly perceived as being harder work for infants. This is categorically untrue as bottle feeding actually causes more physiological stress. If an infant is not physiologically stable enough to complete a breastfeed, then they are also not stable enough for a bottle feed which in fact is likely to be more stressful for them. Bottle feeding is not 'easier' for infants. Babies do not use up more calories breastfeeding, and if they do come to have a preference for bottle feeding rather than breastfeeding this is usually due to flow rate preference, rather than the child demonstrating that bottle feeding is less work. Since we would not say that sucking on a pacifier uses up calories, we should not be suggesting that non-nutritive suckling on a breast uses up calories either.

Infant fundamentals for feeding

So many aspects of feeding we assume, or take for granted, may be the fundamental stumbling block for a child with medical complexity. For example: an infant needs to be able to achieve a seal around the breast and nipple. They need to be able to maintain that seal, and effect negative pressure. To do that, they need an intact palate, normal reflexes, good nerve function, and tongue mobility. They need to maintain breathing and oxygen saturations during feeding and avoid aspiration with a safe swallow. They need to be able to effectively remove milk, sustain the latch and not slip off. They need good muscle tone to maintain head control, jaw movements and mouth and tongue movements. The infant also has to be able to stay awake and alert long enough to be able to complete a feed and take in adequate calories, and the energy they consume must be greater than the energy they expend to remove milk. Finally, once they have transferred milk, they need to be able to digest and metabolise it.

It's probably quite clear now that with all those fundamentals that healthy babies can usually rely on, there are many infants for whom several aspects of the feeding process would be very difficult, which is what we will turn to from Chapter 4 onwards.

Test yourself:

1. What triggers the onset of copious milk production?
   a. Frequent infant feeding.
   b. Domperidone.
   c. Genetic factors.
   d. The delivery of the placenta.

2. What factor will downregulate milk production?
   a. Maternal fatigue.
   b. The degree of milk removal.
   c. Having small breasts.
   d. Tandem feeding.

3. Breastfeeding is harder work for babies than bottle feeding?
   a. True/False.

(All multiple-choice quiz answers can be found at the end of the book, just before the resource section.)

Chapter 3

Common Breastfeeding Challenges

Not all infants and children with medical complexity have hugely complex feeding challenges. Many of them experience common breastfeeding challenges as well - which let's face it are never fun but may be even more stressful in the context of child illness and hospitalisation. It would be easy to think that the degree of breastfeeding difficulty and the level of medical complexity were somehow correlated but in fact this is not always the case. It is true that children with serious illnesses do have unique challenges, which we will return to later, but this does not mean that common problems are not also experienced. Certainly, many mothers have told me that if their child was older and breastfeeding was more established, they seem to experience fewer technical breastfeeding challenges, and more institutional barriers. Other common problems include difficulties with pumping or acute breast fullness. This chapter will review some of the risk factors for breastfeeding challenges, some common infant feeding problems, when to refer for further assessment, maternal breastfeeding challenges and some sources of support.

Risk factors for feeding difficulty

There have been several studies which have explored potential risk factors for feeding difficulty. While feeding is a two way and relational process, some risk factors are specifically related to either the infant or the mother.

Infant related risk factors include prematurity, delayed first feed, facial anomalies, infrequent or ineffective feeding, infants with medical complexity or illness, and infants born to diabetic parents (Genna, 2016; Wambach and Spencer, 2019). There is some evidence that all forms of intrapartum pain relief and birth complications can cause some level of sleepiness or difficulty in newborns (Brown and Jordan 2013; Brimdyr et al, 2015), although this does need more research.

Other risk factors include combination feeding, and the 'top up trap' – the more top ups and bottles infants receive, the lower the maternal milk supply, and the bigger the impact on infant suckling at the breast. Finally, both tongue tie and jaundice are also related to infant feeding difficulty, although there are huge degrees of scale with both conditions (Flaherman et al, 2017; Choo et al, 2020; LeFort et al, 2021).

If you suspect tongue tie in an infant, the child should be referred to an infant feeding specialist with expertise in assessing and treating tongue tie, or an ENT doctor who provides a tongue tie clinic. Tongue tie is a subjective diagnosis defined by restriction in tongue mobility that affects feeding. Sometimes with skilled support, an infant may be able to breastfeed effectively enough to avoid frenulotomy. Other times, if certain factors seem to collide (very firm or fibrous breast tissue, flat nipple, baby with low tone) – even what subjectively looks like a frenulum with a reasonable degree of stretch and movement may be very difficult to feed with. An assessment of the tongue function and breastfeeding efficacy is required to determine the suitability of frenulotomy (Genna, 2016). There is currently no evidence to support the surgical release of lip or buccal ties although there is considerable debate and contention about this, and there are variations in opinion and practice by country (LeFort et al, 2021).

In terms of maternal factors, the onset of lactogenesis II can be delayed by a number of known challenges – such as diabetes of any kind, higher BMI, certain endocrine dysfunction, and retained placental fragment – since lactogenesis II is triggered by the drop in progesterone caused by the detachment and birth of the placenta.

Other risk factors include poor social support, a very long, difficult or operative birth. Another risk factor is extreme exhaustion – it is not the fatigue per se that is a risk factor, but the well-meaning interventions that often go alongside this – such as combination feeding. Postpartum haemorrhage can sometimes cause a drop in blood pressure which if significant, can cause a pituitary necrosis due to blood loss and hypovolemic shock. Although this is unusual, it will hinder the milk production. This condition is called Sheehan's Syndrome and requires specialist lactation input as well as assessment by a doctor as there are other consequences of Sheehan's besides lactation effects (Quandt et al, 2020).

Intrapartum IV fluids can cause both oedema and difficulty with latching, as well as excessive infant weight loss as they excrete the additional fluids, which can lead to a cascade of intervention including the introduction of formula (Giudicelli et al, 2020).

While it is perfectly possible to breastfeed with inverted or flat nipples, they can pose a greater challenge and some studies have found that this is a risk factor for feeding difficulty, often alongside higher maternal BMI (Mangel et al, 2019). From experience this may depend on the combination of nipple elasticity, breast fullness and infant oral anatomy. Some mother-baby pairs seem to struggle more than others, depending on the combination of these factors.

Finally, sometimes there are anatomical and physiological problems related to the structure and function of the glandular tissue of the breast and the innervation of the breast. For example, a history of breast reduction surgery, top surgery, or nipple surgery, as well as chest drain placement and chest trauma. These can damage both the nerves and milk ducts, supplying sensation and feedback to the nipple. Both breast reduction surgery and having a primary case of breast hypoplasia (under-developed breast tissue) is also a risk factor for primary low milk supply. While these are more unusual scenarios, experienced lactation supporters have often come across rarer breast or endocrine conditions, which is why collaborative working with more experienced colleagues can be so beneficial.

Common problems

As I mentioned earlier on, normal and natural does not necessarily mean easy. It is common to run into various challenges, for example:

Mother	Infant/child
Painful nipples	Poor weight gain/faltering growth
Localised redness or swelling in the breast	Reluctance to feed or sleepiness
Breast lump	Difficulty feeding
Low supply (assumed or actual)	Tongue tie

This is why it is important to be able to identify these challenges and refer to the most appropriately qualified professionals for additional support. Challenges such as engorgement (overly full breasts which can become pathologically inflamed if milk is not removed), blocked ducts (an inflammatory response to obstructed milk within the milk ductal system), nipple pain, thrush (candida) and mastitis (breast infection) can all be highly unpleasant for the parent, and in some cases can cause significant illness, so prompt attention should always be sought from a medical professional, alongside skilled feeding support (Amir et al, 2014).

These problems almost never warrant cessation of breastfeeding, but if incorrectly managed can be a risk factor for premature weaning. There are also many infant related problems – including infant sleepiness and difficulty latching.

Whatever the problem, remember the golden rules:

1. Keep the baby fed, preferably with their mother's own milk, or if available, donor human milk, or infant formula.

2. Secondly, protect the milk supply – if milk is not removed, milk synthesis is down-regulated and this can be more difficult to manage the longer it goes on.

3. Finally, work out the underlying cause to target the most appropriate solution so that it can be addressed, alongside preserving the milk supply and keeping the baby fed.

4. Maintain parent-infant connection and bonding – when feeding difficulties are experienced, it is especially important to encourage activities that are nurturing, and also consider self-care.

How breastfeeding challenges may lead to poor weight gain and breastfeeding cessation

In many cases, mastitis, engorgement or nipple trauma have identifiable triggers that can be rectified to prevent recurrence. Shallow attachment for example, tends to lead to a cascade of symptoms, including nipple trauma, blocked ducts, engorgement and mastitis in the mother and low weight gain and fussing in the infant. Because these difficulties are so stressful (and urgent - in the case of poor infant weight gain) there is often pressure to 'fix' the problem quickly. Without skilled support, this often translates into feeding formula in a bottle, often with reduction or cessation of breastfeeding. While bottle feeding and formula may address a weight and nutrition problem, breastfeeding challenges cannot be fully resolved with bottle feeding, and also all the immunological properties are lost.

Breastfeeding cessation or combination feeding is appropriate if it is the parent's choice, but about 80% of parents who stop breastfeeding in the first six weeks are genuinely not ready to (Infant Feeding Survey, 2010). The sad thing is that most mothers probably have the potential for an appropriate milk supply, and may just need some skilled breastfeeding support to finesse the attachment or overcome challenges.

When assessing a breastfeeding mother-baby pair, you will need to observe the infant for signs of adequate intake. The only robust signs of insufficient milk intake are poor weight gain and inadequate output. Frequent feeding, cluster feeding, and a dislike of being put down are all normal infant behaviours.

Plot the infant's weight in their personal child health record (PCHR) or appropriate WHO growth chart, ask about nappy output, and refer for paediatric review if the child is uninterested in feeding, has a fever, presents with reduced urine output, seems unwell, has lost weight, or has signs of dehydration. Also refer children who are apparently feeding well and transferring milk, and yet not gaining weight as expected, since these children may have underlying conditions that have not yet been identified. See https://www.nice.org.uk/guidance/ng75 for more information about faltering growth.

There are many different potential complications of the breast or nipple that can arise during the postnatal period. Not all are directly related to breastfeeding. Some may involve both the child *and* mother. For example, a poorly positioned infant will cause pain and discomfort in the mother, but also may lead to inadequate milk intake in the infant. An assessment by a suitably qualified breastfeeding professional is appropriate, alongside medical management of acute breast or nipple pathology.

Breast complications and pathology

Clinical finding	Possible aetiology
Nipple pain during and after feeding, with nipples that are misshapen, cracked, bleeding or blistered	Shallow attachment at the breast. Requires skilled breastfeeding support
Sudden onset of unilateral breast pain, with skin colour changes, localised heat and a firm area	Mastitis, often secondary to poor attachment at the breast, though not always. Take care when assessing Black and Brown-skinned mothers as they may not have the erythema that many texts describe. Mastitis requires prompt treatment to prevent serious complications such as abscess and sepsis.
Breast lump, with or without pain	There are many causes of breast lump, from galactocele and blocked ducts to breast cancer and abscess. Depending on clinical findings and history, consider referral to a breast clinic.

Clinical finding	Possible aetiology
Nipple discharge	Nipple discharge can be related to various breast pathologies, including mammary duct ectasia, rusty pipe syndrome, papilloma, cancer and cysts. The colour of the discharge and nature of the symptoms will help to pinpoint the cause.
Dry skin	Eczema or psoriasis of the nipple is not unusual, particularly if the mother has a history of eczema. Some mothers are sensitive to laundry detergents, or soaps, as well as foods their older child has eaten.
Sudden onset of shooting nipple and/or breast pain after a period of pain free feeding, accompanied by white plaques inside infant's mouth, cheeks, lips and tongue	Consider candidiasis (thrush). The pain from this is easily confused with pain caused by shallow attachment or poorly fitting breast pump funnels, so expert breastfeeding support is recommended.
Other nipple pain	There are many causes of nipple pain, such as vasospasm, fissure, Raynaud's phenomenon, pregnancy, milk bleb, and psychological causes including abuse.

Diagnostic Tests/Investigations

Appropriate tests depend on the differential diagnosis.

Differential diagnosis	Possible tests
Breast pathology including suspected cancer	Biopsy, mammogram, ultrasound
Mastitis	Consider sending a sample of breast milk for MC&S. Also consider underlying breast pathology and resistant strain infection

Differential diagnosis	Possible tests
Candidiasis of the nipple/ breast	Swab the nipples and infant's mouth for evidence of fungal infection
Poor weight gain	Review weight, breastfeeding assessment, refer for specialist feeding support, paediatric assessment, endocrine referral and blood tests to rule out hormonal causes

Most mothers benefit from peer support, breastfeeding drop-in groups, online support and sources of good information and reassurance (Thomson and Trickey, 2013; McFadden et al, 2016; Trickey et al, 2018; Regan and Brown, 2019), irrespective of whether they have an underlying breast pathology. Remember that many mothers who stop breastfeeding before they intend to experience disappointment and grief (Brown, 2019). It is therefore important to listen, support and encourage, as well as refer to the most appropriately qualified professional. Most breastfeeding problems can be overcome with the right treatment and support.

Mastitis spectrum

Mastitis is now thought to be part of a spectrum of breast pathologies resulting from inflammation and oedema (Mitchell et al, 2022). It can be severe and requires prompt attention. Breastfeeding should not be discontinued, including from the affected breast. Simple measures such as rest, simple analgesics, hot and cold compresses, warm showers, fluids and continuing to breastfeed or express milk from the affected side are appropriate if the mother is haemodynamically stable and not immunocompromised. Massage is increasingly considered to be unhelpful in acute mastitis as this can worsen inflammation.

If simple first line treatment is not working, or the mother's condition worsens within 12-24 hours, then antibiotics are indicated. Flucloxacillin 500mg qds (4 times per day) for 10-14 days is the standard treatment.

If mastitis is recurrent, send a sample of breast milk for microscopy, culture and antibiotic sensitivity (MC&S), refer for specialist breastfeeding support, and consider alternative diagnosis, including breast cancer.

If the mother has signs of sepsis or the infection is progressing rapidly, arrange for hospital admission. The child should be allowed to remain with the mother if desired, with additional support in place to care for the child if the mother is too unwell. If the mother has an abscess, arrange hospital admission and review by a breast surgeon.

For all breast pathology that is suspicious, arrange a 2-week wait referral. For breastfeeding challenges where infant health or weight are compromised, arrange for paediatric review, alongside specialised lactation support. See: https://cks.nice.org.uk/topics/mastitis-breast-abscess/management/management-lactating-women/

Complications of breastfeeding difficulties depend on the underlying pathology. Certainly, breast infections can cause mothers to become systemically unwell, and urgent attention is appropriate.

Many symptoms of breast conditions overlap, which can cause a delay in the correct diagnosis and right treatment. For example, inflammatory breast cancer may be misdiagnosed as mastitis, and sadly I have supported several women who have had this experience. Breast abscess can present initially as a simple blocked duct and quickly escalate. It is therefore important to arrange to review the mother to ensure any treatment is effective. If you are unsure, escalate to a senior colleague or lactation specialist.

Infant signs that indicate further assessment is needed

Ultimately, the only definitive signs of low milk intake are:

- poor weight gain, and
- inadequate urine and stool output.

However, there are plenty of other warning signs – including painful feeding, scant, concentrated 'brick dust' urine (which looks like specks of orange in the infant's nappy) after day 2. Infrequent stools, or stools that have not turned yellow by day six at the absolute latest are also a red flag (Spangler and Wambach, 2014). Babies should wake spontaneously for feeds – if they consistently need to be woken - they should be evaluated.

While a fussy baby after occasional feeds is normal, if a baby is fretful after every single feed, this may indicate a problem, as could pathological engorgement – which indicates that milk is not being removed effectively and milk stasis is occurring. If you remember, the rate of milk synthesis is related to the degree of breast fullness, so if the breast becomes very full, and hard, the rate of milk synthesis will slow or even stop, putting the parent at risk of losing their milk supply.

A baby who cannot latch at all needs evaluation. It could be that there is a fundamental problem with the infant's ability to feed, including a medical problem, or perhaps the parent and baby just need to be shown a different approach. The first recommendation is normally to place the baby in skin-to-skin contact and allow the infant to attempt to self-attach. Since infants utilise their innate feeding reflexes as well as their sense of smell to locate and attach to the breast, this is sometimes all that is needed. Occasionally if an infant is struggling, or there are additional challenges, making a breast 'sandwich' to create a firm 'ledge' for the infant to grasp can help. For other babies, although this should not usually be the first strategy to try, careful use of a thin silicone nipple shield can *sometimes* be effective, though this should always be with informed consent, as it can be hard for some babies to wean from.

Sleepy babies can fall into breastfeeding difficulty if they either do not wake frequently enough for feeds, fall asleep before they have consumed sufficient milk, or are too sleepy to feed effectively. One common reason for sleepiness in the early days is jaundice. Infant jaundice is common and usually resolves spontaneously. However, there are different broad classifications of jaundice:

- Jaundice associated with optimal feeding and normal infant behaviour and alertness, normal weight gain and no pathological symptoms is physiological and usually resolves spontaneously.
- Jaundice associated with suboptimal feeding may result in an infant who becomes dehydrated, experiences faltering growth and becomes systemically unwell. It may require both phototherapy as well as feeding support.

- Jaundice that is associated with pathological symptoms of liver disease requires urgent evaluation by a paediatrician.

If serum bilirubin concentrations exceed the treatment threshold, then phototherapy is usually recommended. The most up to date guidelines suggest that phototherapy breaks of up to 30 minutes for breastfeeding do not affect the efficacy of phototherapy for jaundice (Sachdeva et al, 2015; Flaherman et al, 2017). There is usually no need to separate mothers and infants, or interrupt breastfeeding, although if infants are too sleepy to feed effectively, they may need to receive expressed breast milk via a nasogastric tube, syringe or bottle. Current guidelines also do not recommend routine IV fluids unless there is evidence of dehydration or hypernatraemia.

Why it matters if breastfeeding is painful

There are two main reasons why optimising the child's attachment / latch is critical. One is to reduce pain for the mother, and the second is to maximise milk intake. Breastfeeding problems often affect both infant and mother simultaneously, and painful feeding is no exception. Fundamentally, if the feed is painful, the mother is less likely to continue to breastfeed, and therefore the infant is less likely to receive human milk. But beyond that, breastfeeding problems may be the underlying cause for some admissions, including faltering growth, jaundice and dehydration. Fixing the problem of undernutrition without addressing the cause is disempowering for the mother and may lead to premature breastfeeding cessation.

Painful feeding may also indicate that an infant has some problems achieving an effective attachment or completing a feed. These are signs that further assessment is needed, to rule out dysfunctional suck and tongue tie. Finally, painful feeding is often associated with shallow attachment. If the infant does not have enough breast tissue in their mouth, they may not be able to feed effectively and efficiently, meaning they get less milk, it takes longer to get that milk, they may not be able to drain the breast well, they will have to work harder to get milk, and may need to feed more frequently.

While frequent feeding is not on its own a sign of poor milk transfer, in the context of an unhappy baby, who is struggling to gain weight, and a mother who is in pain, it often points to a shallow latch. The solution is to correctly position the baby and therefore deepen the latch, which often solves most of the problems.

Some quick tips to make feeding less painful:

- Recommend the mother leans back – gravity helps to 'hug' the baby towards the breast, and this usually causes the infant to relax their jaw, and extend their tongue more easily.
- Try to avoid pressing on the back of the infant's head – this tends to confuse infants and can interrupt their feeding reflexes.
- Allow the infant to use their hands – they need them for balance and stability, and also use their hands to massage the breast which stimulates milk production.
- Try to support the infant to have their face touching the breast – in this way, they can use their rooting reflex to locate the breast.
- Suggest that the mother wriggle and squirm around to try to find a more comfortable position.
- Try to make sure that the infant's head and hips are in alignment. If the infant must turn their head to the side to feed, this makes it much more difficult for them.
- Some practitioners teach 'nose to nipple'. This can be helpful for some people to remember that infants need to be positioned asymmetrically for feeding, but in practice, many experienced lactation supporters find that a prescriptive approach can be confusing for parents. You could, instead, recommend that the infant's face is touching, and that the child leads with their chin.

If the infant is positioned with their mouth opposite the nipple, they tend to end up with a shallow attachment, which is both painful for the mother and ineffective for the infant. If the infant is allowed to self-attach, they usually find the right spot without help, as long as their face is touching the breast. However, in more 'mother-led' positions, such as where a mother is seated in an upright chair, this can be harder. In those positions, mothers may need support to position their baby asymmetrically, with the nipple between the upper lip and nose, allowing the child to tip their head back and gape.

Incidentally, positioning infants for comfortable feeding can be harder in the hospital environment. Mothers often tell me that they found it very uncomfortable to feed in hard plastic chairs, or the high-backed chairs with armrests which always seem to be in the way. Some mothers find it more comfortable to feed while lying down, which is harder if the parent bed provided is flimsy, narrow, or not fully flat. It's also harder to breastfeed sitting up in bed without enough pillows, especially with the older style beds that do not have electronic adjustable mattresses. It's hard to believe in this day and age that these relics still exist, but many parents have told me that they were only provided with an ancient hard hospital bed that was unadjustable.

Occasionally, you may need to throw out preconceived ideas about ideal positioning when a baby or child comes your way who has significant medical challenges. Some examples of when classic breastfeeding positioning teaching may miss the mark are:

- Infants who have orofacial anomalies. Sometimes children with high palates, cleft lips, recessed chin or jaw, or nasal malformations need creative adaptations. Don't be scared to think outside the box. I have found, for example, that some children with suboptimal tongue function and high palate seem to do better with a more central mouth to nipple position that would usually make me cringe.

- Children who have low tone sometimes need more head and neck support in order to remain attached to the breast. Again, while this is not suitable for most children, there are some scenarios where purely infant-led attachment may not work, and the infant may waste precious calories trying to maintain head and neck posture. There is a time and place for a mother or helper to intervene, and a time to let the infant try for themselves.

- Children who need respiratory support sometimes cannot be positioned nose to nipple either for very good reasons. If they are receiving high flow nasal cannula oxygen or continuous positive airway pressure they may still be able to feed orally, but it may require some alterations in position to make this work. They may also need shorter and more frequent feeds, and mothers may need support to work out whether to offer the same breast two feeds in a row, or alternate. This is likely to be an individual scenario for each mother-child dyad.

- Children with large wounds, drains, stomas, ports and PEGs, cannulas and central lines or implanted devices. These children sometimes cannot turn their head or body comfortably. Insisting on textbook positioning is likely to make breastfeeding inaccessible for these dyads and instead, a creative and adaptive approach may be necessary.

The bottom line is that each dyad needs to be viewed as unique, with their own strengths and challenges to overcome. No two children with the same conditions are the same, and their mother's anatomy will also be different. Working out what works - given the anatomy and specific issues for a mother and child - will enable you to provide nuanced, individualised care that meets their needs.

Importantly, positioning for comfortable feeding can sometimes be very subtle, and even very experienced breastfeeding supporters sometimes need to call for reinforcements – there is no shame in this. Sometimes someone else's perspective and fresh eyes will see something that can be improved for a family. Never be shy about reaching out to more experienced lactation colleagues for support to finesse the attachment.

Where to find support

Some of you may be well equipped to support the lactation needs of the families you serve. For some, this section has been revision and you would feel confident helping mothers and infants with these common difficulties. For others, this section may be new information and you would not be expected to be able to proficiently handle all of these problems. Rest assured, your encouragement goes a long way for a struggling family, alongside knowing who to refer the family on to for more specialised support.

In the UK, the first professionals that families usually encounter for feeding support are their midwife, health visitor, GP and possibly a paediatrician if the family are accessing private healthcare. According to the World Breastfeeding Trends Initiative, the amount of training these professionals may receive is patchy and inconsistent – they may be highly trained and very experienced, or they may not be (Gupta et al, 2019). My own research has found that most professionals receive less than two hours of training as part of their undergraduate training. BFI accredited maternity, neonatal and health visiting services will have up to two days of training, but knowledge, experience and skills are still variable. Of course, motivated individuals may undertake further independent training but this is patchy and inconsistent.

Parents are also able to access peer supporters and breastfeeding counsellors in some areas, and there are sometimes free drop-in clinics, but again, services around the country vary. There are relatively few IBCLCs in the UK compared with the US where they are more integrated into the health care team. However, some families do access support from an IBCLC either because the IBCLC also happens to also be a nurse, midwife or doctor, or they are accessed via a voluntary or private service. There are also several breastfeeding helplines and I run a free support group on Facebook for parents breastfeeding their medically complex child (*Breastfeeding the Brave*).

If you are concerned about tongue tie, in some areas there may be an NHS tongue tie service, or you could contact the Association of Tongue Tie Practitioners (ATP) should you need to find a health professional who can divide tongue tie. In some countries, tongue tie is only divided by a medical doctor.

There is also a growing body of fantastic medical professionals who are really invested in optimising breastfeeding. They all have websites and Facebook groups and are a brilliant source of support, resources and networking. I highly recommend the *Hospital Infant Feeding Network*, *Breastfeeding for Doctors* and the *Academy of Breastfeeding Medicine* where you will find several well-researched clinical protocols for many, varied situations.

There are several pharmacological resources as well. The '*Drugs in Breastmilk*' email service established by Wendy Jones at the Breastfeeding Network, as well as the *UK Drugs In Lactation Advisory Service* (UKDILAS), *Lactmed* and the *Lactation Pharmacist*. These resources are all listed in the appendix.

As I have mentioned, the level of experience as well as the depth and breadth of training varies hugely between individuals, depending on what training they access. Families should be encouraged to keep asking for support if they cannot find resolution to their problem, but it is also part of everyone's responsibility to understand and acknowledge when a problem is outside their scope of practice or skill set and refer on so that families do not have to keep chasing round trying to find answers.

Test yourself:

1. What is a reliable sign of insufficient milk intake?
   a. Nipple pain.
   b. Jaundice.
   c. Cluster feeding.
   d. Poor weight gain and scant output.

2. A mother exclusively breastfeeding her 4-week old infant presents with a fever over 39C, chills, tachycardia and a throbbing right breast. She has been on flucloxacillin for 48 hours with no improvement and feels acutely unwell. Which is the correct approach?
   a. Advise the mother to go home, rest, drink fluids and take ibuprofen.
   b. Recommend immediate cessation of breastfeeding.
   c. Add in a second antibiotic such as co-amoxiclav and arrange to review her tomorrow.
   d. Arrange for hospital admission.

3. Which of the following are risk factors for feeding challenges?
   a. Diabetic mother.
   b. Poor social support.
   c. Combination feeding.
   d. All the above.

Chapter 4

Why feeding sick children is harder

Many types of feeding can be more difficult when a child is sick or has a medical complication. This includes breastfeeding, bottle feeding, tube feeding and solid foods. But why is this? It may be because of physical or anatomical challenges, but there are many systemic and organisation challenges which add to these difficulties.

Infants and children are cared for in a variety of clinical environments that are not always integrated. Maternity, neonatal and paediatric units, while all caring for children potentially of overlapping ages, are different clinical settings. Maternity and neonatal units may be physically linked or nearby, though they usually have separate nursing and midwifery staff and separate infant feeding teams. By contrast, paediatric wards are often geographically, managerially and organizationally separate from both maternity and neonatal units. Some hospitals do not have all three directorates in the same building. Allied health professionals such as occupational therapists (OTs), speech and language therapists (SLTs), dietitians and physiotherapists usually work across both neonatal and paediatric units though they may have a sub-specialist interest that means they are primarily located in one department. Similarly, doctors often work across all paediatric and neonatal wards, though, once again, some sub-specialist consultants may be primarily situated on one ward or department - for example neonatology or paediatric intensive care unit (PICU). By contrast, nursing staff usually work on one ward. They do not work across multiple wards, but form part of a familiar team on a ward.

Nurses also form a diverse team. Midwives working in the maternity unit may either have an adult nurse background or come from direct entry midwifery training. They usually have no explicit training with older babies or children. Nurses working on the neonatal ward may come from either adult, paediatric or midwifery backgrounds. Nurses on the paediatric ward usually have children's nursing training. The only practitioners who would receive breastfeeding training are the midwives and neonatal nurses *if* their unit happens to be BFI accredited or working towards it. You can see how this gets complicated!

Babies born on the maternity ward who deteriorate are usually taken to the neonatal unit, rather than paediatrics. However, while some very young babies are readmitted after discharge home to the postnatal ward or neonatal unit, often these children are admitted to the paediatric ward. This means that the paediatric ward may admit infants who are days old, and yet are considered an entirely separate clinical directorate (with completely different staff) to both the maternity and neonatal directorates.

Admissions to the paediatric setting – whether a general ward, PICU, specialist ward or day surgery unit will include children with a variety of illnesses and conditions. There is one study that found that breastfeeding was severely negatively impacted by admission of young children to the ward with acute bronchiolitis (Heilbronner et al, 2017). We therefore have some patchy evidence that breastfeeding may be more challenging, or difficult to achieve, when children have a disability, condition or illness, but there are no general studies that explore why this is so, or the impact of this on parents.

Across many health care settings – including maternity, neonatal intensive care, health visiting, children's centres and some universities, the BFI UK standards protect and promote breastfeeding through training, audit and culture change (Perez-Escamilla et al, 2016). However, the standards so far have not been written for paediatrics, and there is no baby friendly accredited children's ward or hospital at the time of writing. Staff within paediatrics are not provided with training as standard, and the experiences of parents are not audited with respect to breastfeeding. There has also been no research to ascertain whether or not the current breastfeeding training, provided as part of BFI accreditation and audit, would meet the needs of staff and families caring for medically complex children on the paediatric ward. What works in one clinical setting and with one population cannot be assumed to work as well in another.

Breastfeeding within the paediatric directorate

Breastfeeding may be challenging to *any* mother-child pair, even without any medical complexity. Breastfeeding a preterm or critically sick neonate presents some additional challenges in addition to those encountered by healthy term mother-child pairs. However, breastfeeding medically complex children within paediatrics is a unique scenario. Medically complex children have some of the same challenges as both healthy term, and sick preterm infants, but they also experience additional and different challenges.

It is likely that parents of medically complex children need a different type of support to initiate or maintain breastfeeding that is tailored to the needs of their child. It is also likely that as well as some overlapping similarities with healthy newborns and preterm neonates, there are different challenges associated with breastfeeding the sick or medically complex population, including older babies and toddlers.

Common challenges among healthy newborns and their parents include finding an effective and comfortable position, correcting the latch, establishing supply, and managing common maternal breast and milk supply problems (Walker, 2021). Professionals supporting parents in the newborn period are often able to troubleshoot difficulties such as blocked ducts, mastitis, low supply, and identify tongue tie. New parents also frequently need support and information about realistic expectations, sleep, normal infant behaviour, adjusting to parenthood and optimising their own mental health (Vanguri et al, 2021).

Infants born prematurely are usually taken to the neonatal unit to be stabilised and provided with appropriate clinical care. The shock and trauma of giving birth to a premature infant is profound (Palmquist et al, 2020), and yet it occurs within an environment which is generally supportive and accepting of breastfeeding as the norm. There is a plethora of research justifying the necessity of human milk (Yang et al, 2020) and human milk based fortifier (Grace et al, 2021), as well as preferentially using donor human milk instead of formula for preterm infants to optimise brain development and prevent diseases including necrotizing enterocolitis, and generally reducing the duration of hospital stay. Using donor milk has increasingly been found to support exclusive human milk feeding and can act as a bridge to getting back to exclusive breastfeeding (Kair and Flaherman, 2017). The risk of giving formula to a very preterm infant is indisputable hence breastfeeding, or the provision of donor milk is strongly encouraged to prevent significant bowel disease (Quigley et al, 2019). We simply don't know if donor human milk would prevent significant disease process or complications as there is just no research on this topic. Undoubtedly, parents of preterm and critically sick newborns have additional and different challenges compared with establishing breastfeeding in healthy newborns – such as dealing with enteral feeding, surgery, and respiratory support, as well as setbacks and illness.

However, I would argue that medically complex children in paediatrics present a much wider range of potential difficulties. While there is a significant and established evidence base in support of breastfeeding or human milk feeding for preterm infants and healthy newborns in general, this is not so in paediatrics. Meanwhile, breastfeeding medically complex children is different for many reasons.

Firstly, illness may occur suddenly and unexpectedly. Protecting a milk supply, maintaining milk production, and transitioning back to breastfeeding are completely different breastfeeding scenarios compared to learning to breastfeed for the first time, as is the case with preterm and healthy infants. Illness that occurs after a period of 'normality' presents a different challenge. While sudden or unexpected stress or shock does not 'dry up' a milk supply per se, it can and does have an impact on the milk ejection reflex. Acute or chronic stress raises blood cortisol levels, which inhibits the action of oxytocin (Lawrence, 2022). When infants and children become unwell, have a serious accident or receive a worrying diagnosis, it is highly likely that parents will be anxious and stressed, which may in turn impair their milk ejection reflex. This makes it much harder for them to protect their milk supply by expressing with a breast pump, and requires skilled and sensitive support and breastfeeding counselling to manage, as many mothers become anxious that their milk supply has abruptly 'dried up'. This support should ideally occur within the context of a ward environment that has a culture of supporting, protecting and promoting breastfeeding for all children.

Secondly, prematurity may present many complications and unexpected setbacks, but in general, the course of prematurity is more predictable, with much known about infant responses, reflexes, behaviours and feeding ability at different gestational ages. In paediatrics, infants and children may present with a vast range of acute and chronic illnesses, conditions and disability, at different ages. Their disease or illness trajectory is therefore far less predictable. Children may be admitted to hospital as an isolated event, experience recurrent admissions, or require lifelong care. The different ages and stages of children admitted will also be directly linked to the stage of lactation, with some time points being more critical to the establishment and maintenance of milk production than others.

Thirdly, there are fewer resources, in terms of training, equipment and research, meaning that good quality information is harder to access. There is usually no expressing room, unlike in the neonatal unit, commonly no breast pumps on the ward, and there is no established precedent for access to donor human milk. It is common for healthcare professionals to misunderstand many aspects of normal breastfeeding physiology – leading to inaccurate or misleading advice. There is often intense pressure to measure and record accurate fluid volumes, and direct breastfeeding is sometimes viewed as a hindrance to this. In short, the environment itself is less conducive to facilitating breastfeeding.

Fourthly, children admitted to paediatrics may have breastfeeding complications that are associated with their development. Older breastfed children may breastfeed much more frequently than usual, or indeed may refuse to feed – both of which may cause confusion and frustration, as well as acute breast-related trauma in the case of avoidance of feeding. Holding a distressed one-year-old who is nil by mouth awaiting surgery is a very different experience to comforting a newborn. Trying to encourage a bored toddler to breastfeed, persuade a hypoglycaemic and sleepy infant to feed, or manage a crawling older infant who is in protective isolation are additional and disparate stressors to parents. As well as developmental challenges, it may also be harder to breastfeed older medically complex children due to central and peripheral lines, wounds, drains, percutaneous endoscopic gastrostomies (PEGs), casts, splints or catheters.

Creative positioning may be needed, alongside maintaining their safety and comfort. The furniture is not always conducive to comfortably feeding an older child, or there may be specific clinical reasons why children prefer to nurse in one position. I have spoken to many parents whose children cannot lie on one side due to the position of central venous catheters such as portacaths (implanted devices embedded under the skin and connected to the superior vena cava in the heart) and Hickman lines (another type of central line that is tunnelled from the jugular vein to the superior vena cava and remains external). These lines are typically used for children who require frequent venous access for giving blood, fluid, antibiotics, total parenteral nutrition (TPN) and chemotherapy. Children may also have lines in their scalp, PEGs, surgical wounds or stomas (openings into the abdomen connected to the urinary or digestive system to allow waste - either urine or faeces - to drain into a bag). This sometimes means that mothers end up only using one breast to feed from. Other children have undergone neurosurgery and need to nurse lying down, which can be hard if the bed is not big enough. There are numerous logistical challenges and constraints that are unique to this population, and require creativity and open-mindedness to overcome.

Medically complex children sometimes have unique challenges related to respiratory needs, low or high tone, higher calorie needs, metabolic complications, anatomical problems, pain and nausea. Layering those challenges over their developmental needs, juggling solid food intake, and maintaining the comfort of familiar home routines presents multiple difficulties for families.

Assuming that a mother has overcome the challenges they have experienced with their child, and maintained their milk supply, children who have been tube fed may need or wish to transition back to direct breastfeeding. This is a different clinical scenario to beginning to breastfeed for the first time, as some children may struggle to return to breastfeeding after a long pause. Additional skills may be required to support a mother-infant pair to return to breastfeeding after a pause due to enteral feeding, nil by mouth, invasive procedures, opiate withdrawal, mechanical ventilation or other respiratory support. There are also challenges associated with increased work of breathing or airway compromise.

There is far less literature relating to re-establishing oral feeding after either invasive or non-invasive respiratory support in paediatrics, compared to neonatal populations. The literature that does exist mainly focuses on short term non-invasive respiratory support such as continuous positive airway pressure (CPAP) and high flow nasal cannula (HFNC) oxygen, and this mostly relates to bronchiolitis (Canning et al, 2021). Some studies find that under-nutrition due to lack of enteral feeding is a common problem in children receiving respiratory support in PICU (Slain et al, 2017; Leroue et al, 2017) even though enteral feeding appears to be well-tolerated and shortens the length of hospital stay (Sochet et al, 2017; Shadman et al, 2019). Feeding difficulties and delay in establishing feeding may have long term consequences for growth and nutrition, oral development, sensory integration and parent-child bonding. These difficulties may be as a result of the child's condition, or there may be an iatrogenic cause (Jones et al, 2021). Difficulty establishing or re-establishing oral feeding after surgical procedures have been found to be more common with longer ventilation times (Eggink et al, 2006), thus enteral feeding and respiratory support appears to be interrelated: Lack of feeding is associated with more invasive ventilation and more critical condition, but conversely, children seem to recover faster with earlier oral or enteral feeding.

Clinical 'skill deserts'

Sometimes maternity or neonatal staff will try to offer support to a patient on the paediatric ward. Although covering paediatrics is often not part of their job description, many will see paediatric 'outliers' as an act of compassion, although this is ad hoc, and only if they have the capacity after managing their usual workload and patient caseload.

Maternity staff are often very experienced with supporting the initiation of breastfeeding in the early days, and adept at troubleshooting common breastfeeding challenges. Neonatal staff are often skilled at supporting very small or sick infants, or providing education and encouragement to express breast milk for an infant who is unable to orally feed. However, the reality is that despite these professionals having skill and motivation to help, they may not be experienced with supporting challenges that are unfamiliar to them, or supporting infants and children who are beyond the newborn stage. Professionals may have a huge range of prior experience, or they may be relatively new in post and only have had experience with a specific population. Parents in paediatric wards or PICU can therefore be caught in what I like to call a 'skill desert', with neither neonatal or maternity outreach fully meeting their needs.

To run with the analogy a little longer, sometimes there is an 'oasis'. Certain clinical environments succeed in supporting mothers to breastfeed their children with medical complexity, and value breast milk as part of the child's holistic care. This may be because there is an influential staff member, a charismatic leader, an established culture of support, a training program, or perhaps many members of staff have had a positive personal experience of breastfeeding, which influences the care they are able to provide. Sometimes a member of staff happens to have additional breastfeeding qualifications and is able to provide informal education and support on the ward. These oases are obviously wonderful resources for parents, but until there is a robust and sustainable fully-funded service, with designated substantive feeding expertise located *on* the paediatric ward and mandatory training provided, these oases are vulnerable. If the level of service provision is dependent on staff, this is a precarious situation, as staff can and do move away, become unwell or burnt out (Brown, 2022), take holidays and go on maternity and parental leave. Providing care to breastfeeding families should not be down to luck.

Due to the different challenges, lack of training for staff (Dykes, 2006; Holaday et al, 1999; McLaughlin et al, 2011; Gupta et al, 2019), and less widespread acceptance of breastfeeding in the paediatric setting, it is likely that parents may have unique experiences of breastfeeding on the paediatric ward or PICU. These experiences may be negative, but parents may also be more motivated to breastfeed their sick children.

What about non-clinical lactation supporters?

If it is clear that breastfeeding training is lacking among many healthcare professionals, then would it be logical to utilise the skills of highly trained and experienced non-clinical lactation advocates instead? Well, maybe. Peer supporters, breastfeeding counsellors and IBCLCs are likely to be highly skilled at not only supporting clinical lactation scenarios, but also usually possess good listening and non-directive counselling skills. This is undoubtedly invaluable for parents caring for sick children who are also dealing with their own grief, disappointment or trauma. However, we must be careful with this population group. While nonclinical lactation supporters are a diverse group and I have no wish to imply that everyone has the same skill set, I have heard numerous examples of inappropriate advice or care being offered to families by some lactation advocates who are *not* clinically trained. This is not only potentially dangerous to children who may be unstable, but can also erode trust in clinicians. It's also not fair to place this kind of responsibility on a lactation professional without clinical training. Sick children can, and do, deteriorate very quickly.

There is already potential for a tension to exist between a parent's desire to be on good terms with the clinicians responsible for maintaining their child's safety and not wishing to appear to be the 'difficult parent', while simultaneously being frustrated with their lack of lactation knowledge and skills. Challenging advice given by a clinician that appears to jeopardise breastfeeding may be entirely appropriate. Yet, there may be times when the clinician's knowledge of the child's underlying condition justifies their advice, irrespective of how this affects breastfeeding.

Of course, the problem is that very often, advice is *not* evidence-based, and therefore many lactation advocates are suspicious of suggestions that on the face of it, appear to be draconian, or unsupportive of optimal breastfeeding. There are endless stories of inappropriate feed volume calculations, strict feeding schedules, or a reluctance to utilise skin to skin without any real reason. It is no wonder that many lactation advocates are quick to challenge advice. But equally, sometimes that advice is given to protect the child, and is based on intimate knowledge of their specific disease or condition and their clinical response to the management. Those outside of the clinical environment may only have one piece of the picture, and may be unaware of the other aspects of the child's condition, perhaps only seeing the situation through the lens of a stressed parent.

Although in some cases inappropriate feeding advice is given by clinicians - and lactation supporters rightly want to advocate for the family - knowing *when* it is safe to handle a child, persevere with direct breastfeeding despite some oxygen desaturation, or trust the child to regulate their intake versus micromanage it are important clinical considerations that are sometimes only understood by a healthcare professional.

Many mothers are skilfully supported by nonclinical lactation professionals for less complex or more stable children, but caution is required when a child is unwell, unstable or has an evolving condition. For example, one mother told me that when a nonclinical IBCLC visited her in hospital and tried to support her attempts to breastfeed after a long period of enteral feeding, the suggestion was to position her baby 'nose to nipple'. The baby had been weaned from invasive ventilation onto CPAP, and the poor mother was unable to get her nipple anywhere near her baby's nose due to the large tubing attached to his face. Another mother I supported had previously felt criticised by a breastfeeding supporter for her child's position when she was asking for help. He did not have his head and body in a straight line, but the reason for this (which the lactation supporter did not account for) was that he had undergone a liver transplant and had an enormous abdominal wound that made rotating him on his side uncomfortable. Another mother told me that when her baby was critically unstable and on high frequency oscillatory ventilation (HFOV) she was advised that it was not safe for her to hold her daughter. When she reached out to a local breastfeeding support group this advice was questioned and implied to be uncompassionate and unnecessary (it wasn't). This made her question the validity of the advice she had been given and wonder whether it was in fact correct, which added to her already considerable anxiety at a time that was extraordinarily stressful.

Breastfeeding advice needs to be nuanced for this population. This sometimes means that advice that would justifiably be considered to be undermining breastfeeding is in fact necessary for the overall health and wellbeing of the child. Withholding feeds, restricting fluids, adding formula, disallowing a parent to pick their child up - all of these uncomfortable interventions are sometimes a case of misinformation, but are occasionally required in the bigger picture, even though they are far from ideal. Working out when a health professional is being too conservative or is misinformed, and when they are truly making a recommendation which is clinically pragmatic is not always easy. Until lactation and health professionals can both respect and lean on each other's different skill sets, there may continue to be suspicion. I suspect the answer is joint training and multidisciplinary team-working, particularly utilising those few professionals who are dual qualified clinicians and lactation professionals. It is vitally important that practitioners stay within their scope of practice, but also that they understand the limit of their knowledge and capacity to help. Lactation advocates have huge amounts of skill and are often also deeply empathic. They are therefore in many ways ideally suited to listening to families coping with serious health challenges. It's just that sometimes it will be necessary to defer to clinical expertise. Equally, clinicians need to know when they are out of their depth and defer to lactation expertise.

When healthcare professionals must be involved

Some infants and children will need to be jointly managed by lactation and healthcare professionals. Obviously, in an ideal world, all clinicians would have the skills required to be able to ensure that a child can continue to breastfeed or receive breast milk if this is the mother's feeding goal. However, I'm mindful that this scenario may be some years away and so for many families, there may be some joint working between two professionals rather than dual skilled single professionals.

When it becomes more tricky is if a nonclinical lactation professional meets these medically complex babies and children in the community, either face to face, or online. If the child you are approached about:

- Is under 35 weeks' gestation
- Is suspected to have an unsafe swallow
- Is on many medications or is known to have complex needs
- Has been diagnosed with hypoxic ischaemic encephalopathy (HIE) grade 2-3
- Has a surgical condition that is ongoing
- Has an evolving neurological condition
- Requires respiratory support including home oxygen
- Is enterally fed (PEG or NG)

- Has complex fluid or calorie requirements
- Is losing weight or has faltering growth
- ...Or you just sense something isn't quite right...

...then these children need to be seeing a clinician as well, and any support should be communicated with that primary clinician. Infants and children who are complex, unstable or whose condition is evolving can often deteriorate very rapidly, and it is crucial that they are overseen by a clinician who is aware of their medical history.

Breastfeeding training in paediatrics

A recurring theme of lack of support and insufficient skills and knowledge within health care professionals in the paediatric setting has been identified in literature supporting breastfeeding and lactation. Additionally, much of the breastfeeding education that exists is weighted towards the initiation of breastfeeding for newborns. In lactation circles, there is often additional expertise around overcoming common obstacles with older babies, teaching toddlers nursing manners and so on. However, I would argue that there are *different* challenges with feeding sick older babies and children that are not well covered currently in mainstream lactation training.

Children who are born at full term, or have ever been discharged into the community will probably be admitted to the paediatric unit if they become unwell, or develop a condition that requires medical treatment. The staff these families encounter may have little to no breastfeeding training or knowledge, and the knowledge they do have is unlikely to be standardised across many units. There are likely to be many differences between hospital units, types of professional, and between different individuals with variable levels of commitment to breastfeeding. Therefore, not only do the paediatric staff not necessarily have the skills required to support families, but the neonatal and maternity staff may lack the necessary skills as well, leaving families at risk of not being able to meet their breastfeeding goals.

Many studies have found that medical complexity is associated with difficulty and lower rates of breastfeeding (Lambert and Watters,

1998; Duhn, 1998; Barbas and Kelleher, 2004; Rivera et al, 2007; Colon et al, 2009; Ryan et al, 2013; Banta-Wright et al, 2015; Torowicz et al, 2015; Helibronner et al, 2017; Madhoun et al, 2019; Barros da Silva, 2019; Coentro et al, 2020) and one hypothesised reason for this could be a lack of health professional training and expertise, as well as a lack of designated and specialised lactation support within the paediatric setting. One study (Heilbronner et al, 2017) found that admission to hospital with an acute respiratory infection was associated with reduced exclusivity and duration of breastfeeding. In this study, the average duration of hospital stay was only three days, and breastfeeding modification was unrelated to severity of illness or invasive ventilation. In fact, the most common reason cited by parents for reduction or cessation of breastfeeding was medical advice. Other studies also echo the correlation of health professional advice alongside inflexible hospital routines with reduced breastfeeding (Rivera et al, 2007; Sooben, 2012; Torowicz et al, 2015).

It is likely that there are many factors related to the quality of advice provided by health care professionals, including undergraduate training, post-qualification training, and personal experience and bias. The World Breastfeeding Trends Initiative (WBTi, 2020) identified many risk factors among the training curriculums of health professionals, noting that there are many gaps (Gupta et al, 2019).

Previous studies have identified gaps in knowledge or attitude of paediatric nurses (Karipis and Spicer, 1999; McLaughlin and Young, 2011; Brewer, 2012; Colaceci et al, 2017) but until my health professional survey there was no study that has explored the knowledge base of *other* professionals. This study did not find a significant difference in skills or confidence between different professionals, or even years of post-qualification experience. The only factor that increased the skills and knowledge of professionals was training and breastfeeding qualifications. The more extensive the qualification, the higher the skill score. Pretty obvious you might think, but useful to know all the same. Importantly, this study only looked at health professionals, so any reference to these professionals being peer supporters, breastfeeding counsellors or IBCLCs is *in addition* to their clinical training. The skills of a dual qualified IBCLC cannot necessarily be assumed to be the same for a nonclinical IBCLC. Of course, this usually does not matter for a healthy child, but it may be highly relevant for a child with medical complexity who requires specialised and nuanced care.

Medically complex and unwell infants and children will be interacted with by a range of professionals, including doctors, allied health professionals (physiotherapists, speech and language therapists, dietitians and occupational therapists) and play specialists as well as nurses and health care assistants. Therefore it is important to recognise the role that *all* health professionals play in supporting breastfeeding, not just medical and nursing staff. It is also important to acknowledge that some more motivated parents draw on external sources of support, or have the resources or knowledge to be able to curate their own package of support using creative means. For example, I have spoken to many parents who hire a private IBCLC from the community, or manage to speak to an infant feeding lead from a different department. Others happen to be peer supporters or know a breastfeeding advocate. Some might have access to an established support group that can provide text or phone support. However, all this requires knowledge of the system, motivation, sometimes money and a certain degree of tenacity. Parents who are more vulnerable, speak English as a second (third, or more) language, are less confident, or have fewer sources of social and lactation support, or no financial means to hire private support, are inherently more dependent on whatever support happens to be available (or not available) on the paediatric ward.

Possible clinical reasons for lower breastfeeding rates

We've already established that breastfeeding is quite a complex and fragile process. It's probably no great surprise to you to learn that rates of breastfeeding are even lower among children with medical complexity. Many studies find that breastfeeding duration and exclusivity is lower, and more difficult to achieve among children with a disease, chronic condition or disability.

Initiating or maintaining breastfeeding for a complex child requires a team effort and provision of resources and additional expertise. There is a lack of data about why medically complex children have lower rates of breastfeeding. Despite these children being cared for in a hospital setting, with access to resources, nursing and medical teams as well as equipment, parents frequently report a lack of support for breastfeeding.

This finding is supported by several studies, though relatively few conditions have been studied (Hookway et al, 2021). There are a small number of studies that have explored the challenges of breastfeeding within very specific groups – for instance Down Syndrome (Barros da Silva et al,2019; Colon et al, 2009; Lewis and Kritzinger, 2004). One literature review found that children with Down Syndrome have lower rates of breastfeeding, and required more support (Sooben, 2012). Another study (Rivera et al, 2007) explored the complexities of breastfeeding infants with Spina Bifida, and concluded it was environmental factors and lack of medical staff knowledge that interfered with breastfeeding rather than infant instability after surgery. There have been a few studies that have explored the challenges of breastfeeding babies with cardiac defects (Lambert and Watters, 1998; Barbas and Kelleher, 2004). Torowicz et al, (2015) also studied infants with a congenital heart defect (CHD), noting that the high-stress environment makes establishing and maintaining a milk supply more challenging. There have also been some studies exploring phenylketonuria (PKU) (Banta-Wright et al, 2015) and cleft palate (Madhoun et al, 2019).

However, no study has looked at the challenges in a general sense, or with older babies or toddlers, and therefore it is hard to make recommendations for practice change that would be applicable widely. There is also only one UK study, involving just five participants (Ryan et al, 2013). This is problematic on two levels - firstly, because the UK healthcare system is unique, and there may be challenges that are specific to the systems and structures that exist within the NHS. Secondly, small samples, while often generating in-depth analysis of someone's experience, are limited in their generalisability. In fairness to the authors of this study, they openly acknowledged that it was a sub-sample of the larger data set for a different study, and was not intended to generate broadly generalisable findings.

What is interesting to me about the existing literature is the lack of variation of illness and condition studied. Some of the studies we have available focus on very rare conditions. For example, one study explored the experiences of mothers breastfeeding their child with Rubinstein Taybi syndrome, which has a population incidence of approximately 1:10,000. The other conditions discussed in the literature are Down syndrome, PKU, CHD and Cleft Lip/Palate. While these conditions are extremely important to understand and provide targeted breastfeeding support, some of them are relatively rare. By contrast, when I recruited parents for the Breastfeeding Sick Children in Hospital study, there seemed to be a fairly representative spread of conditions that children usually present to the average UK paediatric ward with.

Conditions

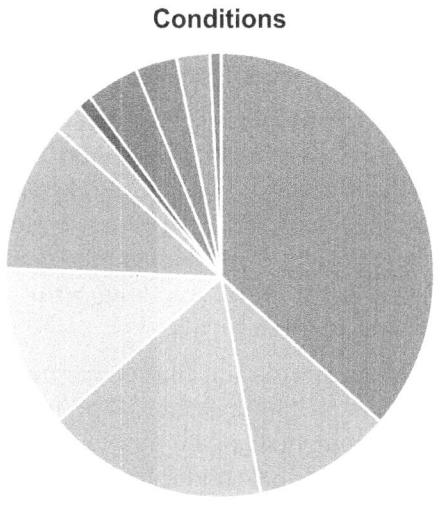

- Lower respiratory tract infection
- Fever/sepsis/infections
- Dehydration/gastroenteritis/ feeding problems
- Cancers
- Neurological/head injury
- Misc
- Upper respiratory tract infection/ airway
- Renal/liver/jaundice
- Cardiac
- Gut/bowel
- Skin and burns

As you can see, from this sample of over 500 children, the vast majority presented to the paediatric ward with an upper or lower respiratory tract infection, acute infection or sepsis. Yet there are no studies that explore how to support breastfeeding in a child with gastroenteritis, meningitis or croup. This is problematic, as clinicians are obviously trying to balance the clinical needs of the child, and without specific breastfeeding clinical skills that help support feeding in a compromised child, breastfeeding sometimes becomes collateral damage.

Sick children and their families not only have to master the skills of feeding, but they also have to deal with a wide range of barriers and difficulties. Infants, children and families may be frightened, in pain, lonely, bored and/or exhausted. Parents may have to deal with separation from other children, financial insecurity and a strange, bewildering parent-child dynamic. There are practical and financial problems, separation from partners and social support, and an entirely abnormal parenting experience (Hookway, 2020).

There are many conditions that you may be aware of - some conditions are transient, such as jaundice and feeding problems. Others have a range of severity – such as respiratory illness and other acute conditions. Just because an illness is short in duration, does not mean it is not severe – for example sepsis, which is not only life-threatening but can also have long term sequelae (health consequences) for some children.

Then there are also chronic conditions that may last for weeks, months or years, such as the complications of prematurity, congenital anomalies, neurodevelopmental and neurological disorders, complex needs, disability, gastrointestinal conditions and metabolic disorders. Other conditions usually present a little later – such as malignancy, autoimmune conditions and acquired diseases.

Broadly speaking, a health condition may either be acute (relatively short in duration, though not necessarily mild), or chronic (a long-term health problem, lasting weeks, months or years). Children may be diagnosed with a health problem antenatally (such as a heart defect), at birth, or at any point in infancy or childhood. Some health problems are inherited (such as sickle cell anaemia and cystic fibrosis), some acquired (such as eczema), and others occur for unknown reasons (such as epilepsy).

The number of children being admitted to hospital is increasing in the UK, with nearly three million children admitted in 2016 (Keeble and Kossarova, 2017). Half a million of these children are under four years old and of these, nearly 40% are admitted via the emergency department. Given that it is normal and common (globally speaking) for children to be breastfed up to the age of two years and beyond, it seems reasonable to expect that breastfed children would be enabled to continue to receive human milk and their families supported to meet their feeding goals. Yet, staff within paediatrics are not provided with training as standard, and the parent's experiences are not audited with respect to breastfeeding.

It is possible that parents of medically complex children need a different type of support to initiate or maintain breastfeeding. This would be tailored to the needs of their child since there are different challenges associated with breastfeeding sick or medically complex children, including older babies and toddlers. Much of the breastfeeding education that exists is weighted towards the initiation of breastfeeding for newborns, and there are different challenges with feeding older babies and children.

When does medical complexity present?

Obviously, the timing of a diagnosis is important. Some families receive a diagnosis before birth. Others know soon after birth. There are also those who find out about their child's condition after weeks, months or even years of their breastfeeding journey being underway. The timing of diagnosis is relevant because clearly, if a prenatal diagnosis is received, this enables some planning, psychological and practical preparation, as well as locating resources and doing some research ahead of time. I have spoken to many parents who were aware of their child's condition antenatally, and managed to set up support, read information to help them overcome challenges, express colostrum antenatally, or find support groups for parents in similar situations. Since we know that good preparation is associated with higher breastfeeding rates, this may buffer some parents, although it is highly dependent on their personal motivation.

A neonatal diagnosis may be quite a chaotic time, as recovery from birth and fielding the combination of congratulations as well as sympathy for a child's diagnosis may be emotionally as well as physically exhausting. A later diagnosis also often means that work, other children and practical issues could be barriers to optimal breastfeeding. In all cases, being able to locate good quality and evidence-based information in a timely fashion is crucial. As you might be aware, breastfeeding compromise sometimes happens quickly.

Especially in the early days and weeks, inaccurate information can spell disaster for the breastfeeding relationship and mental health of the parent.

My PhD research has shown that most paediatric health care professionals seem to be caught on the back foot when they have to quickly find breast pumps or give pertinent information about breastfeeding. Of course, some parents may get lucky and be cared for by a breastfeeding advocate. The mother may have breastfed a previous child, or even be a breastfeeding advocate themselves. However, if the parent does not possess much information about breastfeeding, and encounters a professional who also does not know, then that sets a very different potential outcome before them. I have spoken to numerous parents who have told me that nobody was able to locate a breast pump. Many mothers have been forced to hand express into a sink, or have had to arrange for someone to bring a breast pump from home. One mother told me of her despair when nobody offered her a breast pump during her child's admission, and then the pump she brought from home did not work. Other mothers blame themselves for forgetting to bring their breast pump, assuming it was *their* mistake. Arguably, these mothers should have been proactively offered a pump on admission. It is certainly not their 'fault' that they did not bring a pump from home.

I'm sure many of you have several ideas, as well as your own experience to help you take an educated guess as to how and why breastfeeding medically complex children is harder. The truth is, there really isn't much research though. My systematic review found several potential explanations, including lack of training in paediatrics, and poor provision of lactation support. Unlike maternity and neonatal units, there is almost always no designated paediatric infant feeding lead, or infant feeding team. Then, of course, there are many infant and parent factors, as well as logistical challenges (Hookway et al, 2021). I'm also beginning to hear more and more from parents about specific clinical challenges related to childhood illness beyond the neonatal period that have a direct impact on breastfeeding or maintaining lactation.

The parent experience

Most parents experience a wide range of challenges – including shock, stress, anxiety, depression, frustration, grief and isolation. Many mothers also describe breastfeeding as a buffer though, explaining that it was hard work but worth it, or that they felt committed to preserving this one piece of normality. They also valued the comfort that it brought their children, and one parent felt it helped to restore trust with her toddler after his open-heart surgery.

While it's good to acknowledge the positives of breastfeeding, we must remember how hard illness is for families. Many families describe a hospital admission, or diagnosis of a serious or life-threatening illness as traumatic. For many illnesses, the progression is unclear, or the prognosis uncertain. For some conditions there may be periods of relative normality, followed by sudden flares or relapses which are unnerving and difficult to cope with. Parents often find themselves in a position where they have to drop all the threads of their lives and rush to care for their child, attend hospital or deal with an emergency. For many parents, spending prolonged periods of time on the paediatric ward, away from social networks, friends and their usual routines causes or exacerbates loneliness and depression.

There are numerous difficulties faced by parents when their child is hospitalised – including the difficulty of maintaining connections, travel to and from hospital, and accommodation. Even mundane necessities such as doing laundry can be hugely difficult and stressful when hospitalisation lasts for more than just a few days.

Financially, hospitalisation is hard on families. The costs of parking, travel, entertainment to alleviate boredom, food, as well as loss of earnings from employment are all significant and of course, hit vulnerable families the hardest (Thomson et al, 2016; Beck et al, 2017). There can also be problems around visiting hours and maintaining usual parenting practices, such as bedsharing, and managing to stay connected with partners and other children.

During the Covid-19 pandemic, there were many additional barriers for families, related to visiting and access. Many parents have shared that they were not allowed to have their partner present on the ward, or that a swap with a partner was only allowed once every 24 hours, or every week – there were many seemingly random rules that made it much harder. The rules were also not conducive to supporting breastfeeding. For example, only being able to switch with a partner every 24 hours makes continuing to breastfeed really challenging, and if the parent was tandem feeding their hospitalised child plus a sibling at home, there were often painful and emotive decisions to be made that parents felt unwillingly forced into.

Families not only face separation, but also, life as a parent in the paediatric unit is a profoundly abnormal experience. There is a loss of privacy, the need to parent in an unfamiliar environment, having to adhere to regulations, fixed schedules, protocols, and not being in your own familiar, comfortable and safe space. Social networks are disrupted, and an entire existence has to be conducted in the confines of a 12 x 12-foot square environment (Muscara et al, 2015; Smith et al, 2015; Pelentsov et al, 2015). I have spoken to hundreds of families over the years who have told me how difficult it is to parent in this public way. Everyone on the ward may witness your moment of despair, anger or frustration. Private moments of grief or fury are virtually impossible on an open ward, and some parents have told me that there were no locks on bathroom doors, making showering a really stressful experience. Intensive care and high dependency are often worse, because by necessity, the space is more open in order to carefully observe more critically unwell children. While clinically necessary, this lack of privacy and being constantly visible, I can assure you is stressful. I have spent numerous nights in hospital as a parent. All environments are hard, but resus, high dependency/ intensive care, ED and clinic waiting rooms are the worst. There is nowhere to be human, raw or vulnerable. Even as a nurse with extensive professional experience in these settings, it is unnerving to parent like this.

Lactation related challenges

Then there are the practical challenges of milk production, including initiating lactation, re-lactating in some cases, and maintaining lactation. We mustn't forget that parents may have common and generic breastfeeding problems, in combination with those related to their child's condition. They may need to increase their milk supply to meet the needs of an infant with high calorie requirements, such as infants with cardiac problems or cystic fibrosis, protect it in the case of their infant not feeding effectively during acute illness or surgery, or not being able to be exclusively breastfed, for example, in infants with phenylketonuria. One mother told me that she found it extremely difficult to cope with a blocked duct on the ward, which was probably caused by a suboptimal latch due to the child's respiratory condition. This meant that the child was on and off the breast, and did not feed as well as usual. A blocked duct was not something anyone on the ward could provide advice and support with. Of course, breast and nipple problems aren't much fun at the best of times, but when a mother is stressed and anxious about her child, and in an environment where nobody can help it is much worse.

Parents also sometimes face ending breastfeeding before they wanted to, as well as having to deal with the challenges of being flexible with lactation for an infant who is unable to receive human milk without adaptation, such as those with inborn errors of metabolism, congenital lactose intolerance, or chylothorax. One mother made an informed decision to stop pumping when it became clear that her child would never be able to directly breastfeed. She had persevered with pumping in the hope that one day her baby would get back to the breast, but the child's condition worsened, requiring the difficult combination of fluid restriction, higher calories and ultimately a tracheostomy and long-term ventilation. Breastfeeding was reduced and reduced until it became such a negligible part of the child's diet that it felt like the small amount of milk allowed was not worth the effort it took to maintain. This mother had made so many sacrifices to continue expressing milk that she eventually made an informed choice to slow down the pumping with a view to stopping. The story is a positive one and just shows that when mothers and parents receive compassionate, individualised care, they can be enabled to stop breastfeeding in a way that they feel good about.

These psychological challenges can also affect lactation success. Stress and anxiety can affect the milk ejection reflex, and it can be hard for some mothers to pump or breastfeed their child in a very public place, with pressure to achieve certain volumes. Imagine having to express milk in the paediatric intensive care unit with all the triggering sights and sounds, under the watchful gaze of other parents and professionals, especially if you are the only one breastfeeding. Many parents have told me that vicariously traumatic experiences, such as a child dying in the next-door bed space in the

PICU, were deeply difficult both psychologically, and also practically. One mother described having nowhere else to go to express milk, and yet also felt it was insensitive to continue pumping one metre away from a couple whose child had just had their care withdrawn.

Sometimes, parents are forced to give formula despite having a normal milk supply, due to their child's inability to digest their milk – for example if they cannot tolerate the fat, lactose or phenylalanine in milk. Sometimes infants are fluid restricted or fluid overloaded. They may have very high losses from their stoma, drain, secretions or as a result of vomiting and it is impossible for their mothers to produce the vast amounts of fluids required to replace those losses. Some children have very high calorie needs plus fluid restriction, which means that it is impossible for them to get the calories they need from breast milk, as the correct amount of calories would result in fluid overload. These are really difficult clinical scenarios that require sensitive communication to ensure that mothers do not feel like their milk is irrelevant or unimportant. It's so easy sometimes to focus on millilitres, fluid requirements, calorie calculations and forget that there are human emotions to account for.

Maintaining a milk supply that won't be used by their child can feel very demoralising. It can also be difficult to maintain milk supply due to lack of skin to skin, like one child in my 2019 informal survey who was very unstable after her open-heart surgery and could not be moved for several days. Finally, some parents described having a mixed relationship with a breast pump, describing it as cumbersome, lifesaving, degrading, and essential, sometimes in the same breath. Several parents have told me that they *hated* pumping, that it was purely sacrificial, and never once enjoyed it.

The reality is that children who are seriously unwell face a mind-boggling array of treatments and interventions, many of which will have an impact on their wellbeing, as well as their ability to breastfeed. Children may face surgery, chemotherapy, blood tests, arterial, central and peripheral lines and cannulas, feeding tubes, oxygen, invasive ventilation and CPAP, steroids, drains, IV fluids, transplant, transfusions, scans, x-rays, and numerous different drugs. Many of the children I have had the privilege of meeting and supporting have had more interventions that most adults will endure in their lifetime.

We cannot under-estimate the challenges facing children with complex needs, or their mothers/parents. We also cannot assume that the simple breastfeeding interventions that work for uncompromised children will work in the same way for children with medical challenges. One mother told me that someone suggested she look at a photo of her child to help with her let-down reflex while she was pumping. This is a perfect example of how advice that often works for one population does not necessarily work for another. She told me that looking at a photo of her child who was critically unwell was certainly *not* conducive to optimal milk production.

Motivations to breastfeed a sick child

Breastfeeding is a relationship, providing comfort, nurture, familiarity, connection and love. It's not just about the child, or about the milk. If a child cannot be directly breastfed, this can be a great disappointment to some mothers, who value the close contact as much as the fact that their child is receiving their milk. Many mothers have described profound levels of grief and despair when they have been unable to breastfeed.

Many parents are deeply committed to breastfeeding their child even before they became unwell or received a diagnosis. Some know they will breastfeed before they even become pregnant or make plans around how they will feed their child before birth. It is not a trivial detail. Other parents become *even more* motivated to persevere when they know their child is sick.

Breastfeeding can bring a sense of involvement, purpose, and a feeling of doing something constructive, positive, and normal (Matthews et al, 1998; Scott and Coln, 2002). Others are motivated to continue due to the positive immunological support that their milk provides for their vulnerable infant or child (Smith, 2019). And most parents also describe the reassurance and comfort that breastfeeding brings their child at a scary or difficult time.

Children who are unwell may receive many interventions and treatments, but for many parents, human milk is a significant modifiable factor that is worth fighting for. More research is needed in this area, but children who are breastfed often have reduced severity of illness, shorter length of hospital stay, less hospital acquired infection and fewer complications (Laguna-Cruz and Becina, 2017). This may in turn be related to the active immunological components in human milk, such as macrophages, immunoglobulins, lactoferrin, lysozyme and lymphocytes, which actively ingest bacteria, and support the child with passive immunity (Fuster-Jorge et al, 2011).

So ultimately, for the children who could potentially most benefit from receiving human milk, their families often find that the barriers to continuing to do so are insurmountable – which is why we must do better.

Stories from parents

I conducted an informal survey of parents via social media, asking parents if they wanted to share their story of persevering with breastfeeding through illness. I had over 60 responses. I asked them whether they were supported to breastfeed on the paediatric ward, what would have helped, and there was a section where they could expand their story. Many of the parents wrote several pages detailing their experiences. Here is a selection of the comments I received from the participants of the Breastfeeding the Brave Project in relation to what breastfeeding meant to them at a very hard time. One child had Cystic fibrosis, one had cancer and another had a major cardiac defect and received ECMO (Extracorporeal Membrane Oxygenation):

"When I was allowed to feed him while he was having a cannula changed, it was amazing to watch the needle pierce his skin but see that he didn't even flinch or show any signs of pain."

Fay

"Whenever we were admitted to hospital because he was refusing to eat due to chemo sickness, he would always take milk from me and was less likely to be sick after it."

Georgie

"It was the first time they had let anyone breastfeed on PICU, and I was nervous with all the drains and wires still in place. The nurse and two doctors watched the monitors closely in amazement as his blood pressure went down to normal and his oxygen levels rose.

They couldn't believe it, 'You have magic milk!' they exclaimed.
After that, his recovery was rapid."

Lucy

Parent stories are incredibly powerful, and often speak volumes. I therefore want to share some cases with you to illustrate the importance of breastfeeding to sick children and their families. I'll share some longer stories and images from parents in Chapter 6.

Sophie's story

Sophie began breastfeeding well, but when her son was a few weeks old, he became very fussy at the breast, to the extent that Sophie was considering stopping breastfeeding. She persevered, and sometime later, her baby was diagnosed with a thoracic neuroblastoma. Neuroblastoma is a type of cancer most common in children under five, and it develops from immature nerve cells. He was diagnosed with cancer at just nine weeks old and started chemotherapy at four months. The success story here is that this baby started to breastfeed well once his disease was diagnosed and his chest tumour was removed. He went from being very fussy at the breast to breastfeeding happily, and unlike so many babies who have cancer, he did not need an NG tube, and is now gaining weight faster than ever. Plus – Sophie went from finding breastfeeding frustrating to enjoying it and feeling glad that she can protect his immune system with breast milk while he is immunocompromised by chemotherapy.

Rebecca's story

Isaac was diagnosed with Hypoplastic Left Heart Syndrome at the 20-week scan. Rebecca threw herself into researching what she could do, and how to ensure her breastfeeding journey would be successful. She started to express colostrum in pregnancy, and initiated pumping early on. She actually ended up with an oversupply, but was thankful to have too much, rather than too little. Isaac was able to breastfeed from 10 days old and continued to breastfeed through two of his three open heart surgeries, until he was two and a half years old. Even more remarkably, Isaac never needed any high calorie formula or tube feeding at home. On one occasion as Isaac came round from surgery, he was fussy and unsettled, and nothing could calm him down. Rebecca kept insisting that the fussing was just him communicating that he wanted to breastfeed. They had never had a baby breastfed on PICU before, and eventually, after several conversations with numerous staff members, they went ahead and picked him up to breastfeed. He immediately calmed down and became physiologically stable, to the amazement of the staff watching.

Alice's story

Freya was born at 33 weeks with severe intrauterine growth restriction (IUGR). Alice had been very unwell with pre-eclampsia resulting in an emergency caesarean. Freya was just over 1.2kg at birth and developed necrotising enterocolitis (NEC) at seven days, and all oral feeds were stopped so that her gut could recover. She received total parenteral nutrition (TPN) during this time. At two weeks, the family learned that Freya had cystic fibrosis – a genetic condition where sticky mucus builds up in the lungs, and gut. It makes children much more vulnerable to infections and also prevents them from absorbing all the nutrients from their food. Freya really struggled with faltering growth, and even with a nasogastric (NG) tube, nipple shields to help her achieve a seal and breastfeeding, she was still struggling to gain weight. At 10 weeks, she was diagnosed with a bile blockage that finally explained why she wasn't absorbing nutrients and putting on weight. Now that she is on the right enzymes and treatments, she is thriving.

Sadly, there aren't always great experiences for parents. In my 2019 informal survey there were a few examples of supportive care, but sadly the vast majority of parents reported a lack of support for breastfeeding. I picked out a handful of their experiences to share with you:

"I was really pressured into giving high calorie formula. I really felt that they just didn't want me to breastfeed. If the dietitian had her way she would have had my baby on full formula feeds."

Harley

"As they needed to measure input vs output it felt to me like breastfeeding was a hindrance to them."

Anna

"I was chastised, in front of others, for breastfeeding. I was told I should 'never have been allowed to breastfeed' as it had 'caused' a lot of my baby's issues. She hadn't read the file properly and had no idea of the history. She never apologised."

Cindy

"All the doctors were extremely unsupportive. They told me I was being 'selfish' because I didn't want him to have formula. I felt so much pressure to stop feeding."

Maha

"Most hospital staff just wanted me to formula feed her as she was so sick."

Jude

While these examples are not representative of everyone's experience, it is important to note that parents continue to experience not just inaccurate information, but also on occasion hostility from staff.

When I consider what parents have told me about the huge variety in responses from staff in paediatrics, I think of it like this - when we 'take the temperature' of support in paediatrics, most parents I speak to describe care that is neutral. While this might sound benign, parents usually do not interpret neutrality or a 'whatever you want is fine' approach positively. They mostly want to be encouraged and to feel like the staff understand how important breastfeeding is to them. When staff on the ward imply that it doesn't really matter - even if their intention is to be encouraging - this is hurtful, particularly when breastfeeding is so meaningful to them or their child.

Many parents tell me that their sense is that the staff do not want to pressurise parents into breastfeeding. This is, yet again, an example of how paediatrics is different from the maternity setting. While some mothers who have just given birth and feel ambivalent about breastfeeding interpret encouragement to breastfeed as 'pressure', in paediatrics breastfeeding may already be established. It isn't the same context at all. If the mother is already breastfeeding then supporting them to continue is not pressurising, but facilitating a parental feeding decision. Although many professionals have kind intentions here, and want to remove any pressure at all from a parent in a stressful situation, it's important to listen to the parents' feelings and wishes.

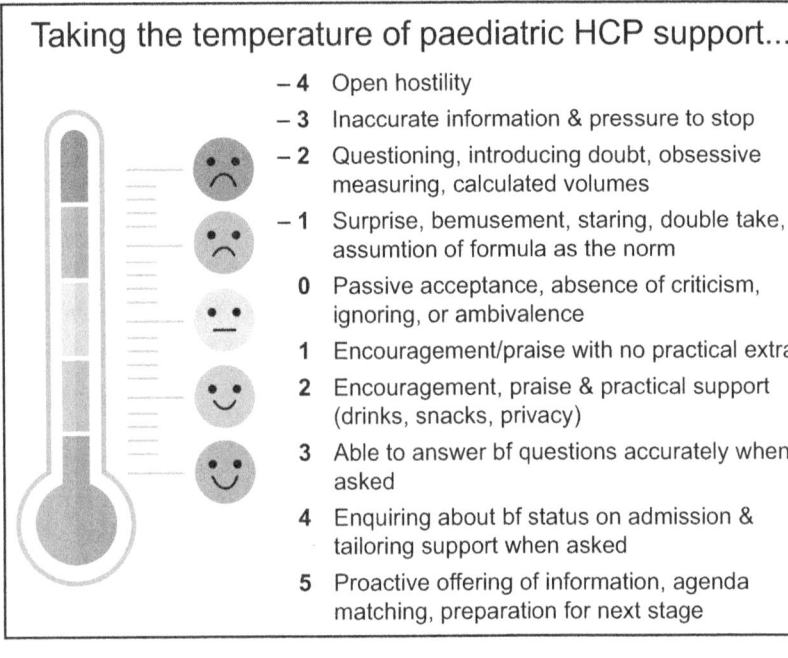

Taking the temperature of paediatric HCP support...

− 4	Open hostility
− 3	Inaccurate information & pressure to stop
− 2	Questioning, introducing doubt, obsessive measuring, calculated volumes
− 1	Surprise, bemusement, staring, double take, assumtion of formula as the norm
0	Passive acceptance, absence of criticism, ignoring, or ambivalence
1	Encouragement/praise with no practical extras
2	Encouragement, praise & practical support (drinks, snacks, privacy)
3	Able to answer bf questions accurately when asked
4	Enquiring about bf status on admission & tailoring support when asked
5	Proactive offering of information, agenda matching, preparation for next stage

If you are a healthcare professional working clinically, I wonder - as you look at that 'temperature' gauge - where you feel your unit sits? Can you recognise professionals you have met within that scale? Do you feel that improvements could be made?

It's important to think critically about your clinical environment (if applicable to you). Remember the skill desert analogy from the beginning of this chapter? You may be an oasis for your unit, but what happens when you are on annual leave, or sick? Does the support offered to families drop from a +4 to a -3? How could you implement a system where care is more proactive, compassionate, protective of lactation and family centred?

Emma's story

The reason it is so important to think about ward culture is that this can clearly affect the experiences of parents. I want to share with you an example of when breastfeeding support was really lacking and led to premature and unwanted cessation. Emma's story is profound, and hugely important. Emma wanted to share her story because – in her words - if it prevents just one person going through what she endured, it was not entirely pointless. Emma's son James had no apparent problems at birth. He breastfed soon after birth, and they were exclusively breastfeeding. At eight weeks, James stopped breathing. He was diagnosed with urosepsis, and a chest infection and was admitted to hospital where alongside breastfeeding, he was topped up with formula down an NG tube. But James's problems didn't end once he recovered. He was diagnosed with laryngomalacia (floppy larynx), as well as severe gastroesophageal reflux disease (GORD) and an unsafe swallow, apnoeas and subglottic stenosis. His weight started to falter, and he was diagnosed with faltering growth. By the time he was a year old he had had 21 hospital admissions, including four HDU admissions, and eight ambulance rides. He had major airway surgery at seven months, and then it all really started to go wrong with breastfeeding.

A video fluoroscopy showed that he was aspirating fluid during bottle feeding, and a speech and language therapist said that Emma had to immediately stop breastfeeding due to his unsafe swallow. There was, sadly, no consideration of whether breastfeeding would have caused the same level of aspiration. Video fluoroscopy cannot assess breastfeeding – it can only measure bottle feeding, so it is like comparing apples and oranges. It is also unclear to what extent aspirating on breast milk is problematic. There is no guideline at the current time to help professionals navigate this unknown area, though many professionals believe that aspirating on small amounts of breast milk is unlikely to cause harm in the same way that formula would. However, despite some compassionate support to immediately stop breastfeeding and reduce milk supply, there were no discussions held with Emma to help her explore her options or risk assess the situation. She felt blamed, humiliated and surrounded by people who didn't care.

Emma told me, *"I was forced to give up the most special thing I had because of people's lack of information and knowledge. He is still poorly and there are more surgeries to come, yet this time I won't be able to comfort him by breastfeeding him. A concept which breaks my heart because when he was poorly that was all I could do for him. It's awful. It's really affected my mental health. It was the best thing I ever did and I don't think I will ever be able to get over what happened."*

Breastfeeding is more than just milk. It is a way of mothering. It's a way of parenting (Brown, 2018). A way of caring. A way of loving. When you take breastfeeding away from a parent, it isn't about removing one type of milk and replacing it with a different type. It isn't even about removing direct breastfeeding and replacing it with a different feeding route. Fundamentally, it removes a parenting tool and can cause grief and trauma (Brown, 2019). This grief is carried for years, or as Emma says, forever.

Test yourself:

1. Which factors related to infant illness may be associated with lactation difficulty?
   a. Inhibited milk ejection reflex.
   b. Lack of health care professional training.
   c. Needing to maintain milk supply.
   d. All of the above.

2. Which of the following interventions is *most* supportive of lactation in medically complex children?
   a. Recommending that the staff bottle feed the child to give the parent some rest.
   b. Ensure parents know that they don't have to breastfeed if they don't want to.
   c. Encourage skin to skin contact.
   d. Explain that breast is best, especially when babies are sick.

3. Breastfeeding is not just about nutrition, but immunologic support, comfort and providing normality.
   a. True/False.

4. Which of the following are valid reasons to breastfeed a medically complex child?
   a. It may be one of the few 'normal' parenting activities a parent can do.
   b. It provides comfort to the parent.
   c. It provides immunological support to the child.
   d. All the above.

Chapter 5

Filling the gap in the current evidence base

One of the problems of healthcare professional competency is that breastfeeding and lactation is not a core clinical subject covered by undergraduate nursing, medical or allied health professional training programs (See Table 1 below). Therefore, training in breastfeeding is patchy and inconsistent, with students currently relying on clinical placement experience and tuition by a clinical mentor on the ward, or needing to supplement their training with post-qualification courses.

The Nursing and Midwifery Council (NMC) Field specific competencies for Children's Nurses (2014) do not specifically mention breastfeeding or human lactation. There are numerous references to competencies that would be indirectly applicable to breastfeeding if the reader chose to interpret them thus, but the only specific reference to feeding is the competency for enteral (nasogastric [NG] and percutaneous endoscopic gastrostomy [PEG]) feeding).

Allied health professionals have standards of proficiency that are available on the Health and Care Professions Council. Speech and language therapist standards (2014) have no mention of infant feeding, nor do dietitian standards (2013), or physiotherapy standards (2013).

Postgraduate medical training is divided into several subspecialties by the General Medical Council (GMC). Doctors who are likely to encounter infants, children and lactating mothers include paediatricians, general practitioners, and obstetricians. The Royal College of Paediatrics and Child Health curriculum (2018) has one mention of nutrition, and it is under the subspecialty of Gastroenterology, hepatology and nutrition, referring to the management of children with complex nutritional needs. The Royal

College of General Practice (2019) curriculum has a few generic references to health promotion and preventative healthcare but no specific statement about lactation or infant feeding. Finally, the Royal College of Obstetrics and Gynaecology (2019) has no discussion of infant feeding or breast care at all, even under the postnatal care competencies.

Table 1: Summary of health care professional competencies relating to infant feeding

Health Care Professional	Competencies that mention infant feeding
Paediatric nurse	Enteral feeding only - not oral
Doctor	No mention of infant feeding
Speech & Language Therapist	Ethical implications for withdrawal of feeding
Dietitian	Ethical implications for withdrawal of feeding
Physiotherapist	No mention of infant feeding

Despite oral infant feeding not being taught as a core competency on any paediatric health professional training, many individuals access further training either privately, or through training budgets within the NHS. There are a variety of courses, both in-person, online, taught and self-paced.

Additional breastfeeding training options

The most commonly accessed training options are one to three day Baby Friendly training, peer supporter training, breastfeeding counsellor training, and IBCLC preparation courses. There are differences in the breadth and depth of these training courses (see table 2), as well as cost, accessibility, and expected career pathways following completion.

Table 2: Summary of differences between training options

	Baby Friendly Training	Peer supporter	Breastfeeding counsellor	IBCLC
Primarily accessed by	Health care professionals	Usually women who have breastfed their child	Mothers who have breastfed at least one child for >6 months	Health care professionals and breastfeeding counsellors
Clinical hours required	None	None	None	1000 verifiable and supervised hours
Assessed by	No assessment, but audit annually in accredited areas (none currently in paediatrics)	Completion of training, DBS check	Short answer questions, scenarios and some courses are also accredited	Meeting pre-requisite standards and 4 hour exam
Breastfeeding training hours	Average 15-18 hours over 2-3 days	Average 16-36 hours over about 12 weeks	2 years training part time	Minimum 90 hours lactation specific education after HCP or BFC qualification
Re-assessment	BFI accredited units require annual audit and training updates. However, BFI accreditation is not currently offered to paediatric units	Most organisations provide continuing education	Varies, but most organisations offer continuing education	Must attend 75 hours of continuing education to recertify every 5 years
Scope of practice	Health professionals utilise their training within the scope of their role	May volunteer in breastfeeding clinics, or have a paid role in a hospital. Refer to health professionals or BFC when necessary	Usually volunteers on a breastfeeding helpline, and also may run breastfeeding clinics. May supervise and train peer supporters	Many work in NHS settings, training roles, others work privately. IBCLCs manage complex feeding issues

	Baby Friendly Training	Peer supporter	Breastfeeding counsellor	IBCLC
Clinical competencies taught	Basic lactation physiology, common breastfeeding problems, attachment and relationship building, supporting expressing, starting solids,	Basic lactation physiology, common breastfeeding problems, how to support expressing, introducing solids, and basic counselling skills	Extensive counselling skills, supporting a range of breastfeeding problems, expressing, supporting parenting	175 competencies including: Anatomy and physiology of lactation, nutrition, endocrinology, infant and maternal pathology and toxicology, psychology, clinical skills, equipment, counselling skills, research, public health
Any information about sick children?	Some common health challenges such as jaundice and hypoglycaemia of the newborn	None	None	Pathology competencies include palate anomalies, some disabilities, metabolic diseases and general response to illness/surgery

Adapted from 'Who's Who in Breastfeeding Support and Lactation in the UK' (Lactation Consultants of Great Britain, 2017) https://lcgb.org/why-ibclc/whos-who-in-breastfeeding-support-and-lactation-in-the-uk/

Baby Friendly training is considered the minimum standard for professionals supporting lactation in clinical practice. In paediatrics this is not mandated at present, a risk highlighted by indicator five of the World Breastfeeding Trends Initiative (2016) though there are some standards being developed.

While it is likely that there are pockets of good practice, the current evidence as well as anecdotal data suggests that this is the exception rather than the rule. Current breastfeeding support provision within paediatrics may be ad hoc, patchy and opportunistic. For example, there may be enthusiasm from certain individual practitioners, but this is not a sustainable model as it relies on the advocacy and influence of that individual. The systems, training schemes, policies and culture of supporting breastfeeding are not firmly embedded in a robust and systemic way, leaving families vulnerable to falling between gaps in services.

What is also obvious is that there is extremely little teaching available about how to modify or adapt breastfeeding for a sick child. The IBCLC teaching blueprint does include some brief theory about clinical conditions - mainly focused on those conditions about which there are studies. As I previously mentioned, there are some studies relating to managing children with cleft lip/palate, congenital heart defect, and phenylketonuria. However, there is not enough clinical detail to equip someone new to these conditions with the skills to overcome these challenges, particularly when some of these conditions are fairly rare. While some strategies can be borrowed from work in the neonatal setting, as I have mentioned, this is not always appropriate, and therefore sick older children often fall between cracks. Sadly, it is not only the children with rare diseases that are falling through the cracks - it's also the children with diarrhoea, chronic wheeze, fever and all manner of common illnesses too.

The current evidence base

When I first set out to undertake a systematic review as part of my PhD, the differences between paediatric, neonatal and maternity feeding issues seemed so obvious to me that I assumed reviewing the literature would be a gigantic task involving sifting hundreds of papers. The fact that I had not come across any significant research up to that point was something I put down to not looking properly (impostor syndrome at its finest here!). I simply assumed that it must be out there, hiding under a different keyword. I started looking for literature in 2019, and was immediately struck by how little research was available.

The inclusion criteria for the systematic review were - all studies written in English, concentrating on parents who were breastfeeding their infant to any degree, in the paediatric setting, that were exploring the challenges of lactation with the medically complex paediatric population. I set no time limits, or geographical limits to the research, as I wanted to establish the existing body of knowledge around the challenges and needs of mothers breastfeeding their sick infants or children in the paediatric setting. The second objective was to identify the gaps in healthcare provision that act as barriers to maintaining breast milk supply and facilitating breastfeeding in the medically complex paediatric population.

My search yielded 786 papers, of which the vast majority were irrelevant to the review. Many studies were clearly focused on the NICU environment or focused on breastfeeding being a preventative or protective intervention against illness. Overall, there were eight qualitative studies, and three mixed methods studies, representing a total sample size of 599. All the studies explored the impact of illness, disability or congenital anomaly on breastfeeding and discussed a huge variation in practice, across different healthcare systems. Some studies also explored the parental experience of breastfeeding through medical challenges. Of eleven included studies, six were conducted in the United States or Canada. There was just one UK based study, which had a very small sample size, and it was notable how few illnesses or conditions were explored.

I identified two parent related themes – one relating to practical and logistical problems, such as overnight accommodation, caring for other children, social isolation, and financial strain. The second parental theme related to stress, anxiety, depression, and some of the impacts of these problems on milk supply.

There were two main infant themes – one relating to infant critical illness, recovery or instability, and the other relating to specifics of the child's condition that were barriers.

There was a specific theme that emerged relating to the provision or lack of provision of lactation support. The sixth theme was about healthcare professionals training and attitudes, and finally, several studies discussed specific equipment, techniques, adaptations and resources that they needed in order for breastfeeding to work, which I will return to later on.

Multi-disciplinary support for families

I genuinely believe that care for families is better when we know exactly who the right person is to involve in a family's care. Not all families require all of these specialists, but many do. A paediatric team that fully values the role of the play specialist alongside the speech and language therapist, or the IBCLC alongside the dietitian. Peer and social support alongside psychological support. It's not just about having a feeding team present on the ward, but fully integrating that with the existing multidisciplinary team.

I also believe that collaborative working does not mean that we all have to know it all. If we could achieve both health and lactation professionals moving towards a greater understanding of the gaps in knowledge, then I'm pretty sure families would benefit. Lactation professionals need more training in the unique needs of sick children, and healthcare professionals need more training in the importance and value of breastfeeding, including how to support families to overcome challenges, and when to refer to specialist and designated lactation support (Hookway, 2020). Those with dual skill sets as both lactation advocates and clinicians are valuable to shape services in the early days as they have unique integrated knowledge that could be shared with the wider clinical and lactation team, and they could be responsible for leading teaching and mentoring less experienced staff for example.

A vision for integrated care – the paediatric infant feeding team

I would love to see designated infant feeding teams led by an infant feeding lead for paediatrics, located on the paediatric ward, and their time ringfenced just for children on the paediatric wards, as well as the outliers in the Emergency Department, PICU, Cardiac Critical Care, Ambulatory Care and Rapid Assessment Units.

I also believe that there should be an Infant Feeding Medical Director post, and Infant Feeding Champions identified among paediatric nurses, health care assistants and allied health professionals. There would ideally be peer support located on the paediatric ward as well, offering practical ideas and strategies, as well as being able to listen to families.

One paper I reviewed specifically identified paediatric peer supporters in the context of learning how to breastfeed infants with Down's syndrome, and found this helpful and validating (Lewis and Kritzinger, 2004). Good transfer planning between NICU and PICU would be beneficial to support those long-term NICU graduates from slipping through the feeding support cracks between neonatology and paediatrics. Sometimes babies discharged from neonatal care require closer monitoring at home, and these children need care from appropriately trained professionals who can identify a clinically fragile or deteriorating child.

Designated paediatric infant feeding training should be mandatory. It is an urgent priority, and should be tailored according to role. Specific, nuanced paediatric baby-friendly standards should be fully adopted throughout the paediatric setting. Training should equip professionals to be able to support parents with the challenges identified in this specific population, rather than assuming that what works in other clinical environments will automatically work in paediatrics.

Finally, it should go without saying that there should be allocated resources for families in paediatrics, including their own supply of breast pumps so these don't need to be begged and borrowed from the postnatal or neonatal wards. There should be a designated, private expressing room with milk storage facilities, and pasteurised donor human milk should be available for certain children who would benefit immensely from the immunologic protection it would offer them.

There is nothing to stop you from seeing how many of these changes you could implement on your unit. It's worth talking to your manager, recruiting other committed and motivated individuals, and making some changes. You may even be able to get funding for equipment, additional training, or resources. Many changes start with one person initiating a cascade of improvement.

Iatrogenic breastfeeding effects

It is perhaps logical to assume that when mothers of medically complex children stop breastfeeding or start combination feeding that this is due to the nature of their infant's illness, or is perhaps more associated with an illness of long duration. Maybe we might think that it is related to incompatible conditions or that it is maternal choice.

Yet, the limited research available does not suggest this, and nor do the experiences of hundreds of families who have reached out to me. Short admissions do not necessarily mean less disruption to infant feeding. Long term admissions are not necessarily related to more disruption, and more severe illness is also not necessarily related to higher levels of cessation or less exclusive breastfeeding. It appears that as soon as a family is admitted to the paediatric ward, there is something about the environment, support, advice and recommendations they encounter which leads to unwanted breastfeeding cessation.

The vast majority of children who present to the emergency room have an acute infection, such as a respiratory tract infection, gastroenteritis or other acute infection. These conditions are less likely with exclusive breastfeeding - in fact about half of all cases of gastroenteritis and a third of all cases of respiratory infections could be prevented by breastfeeding (Victora et al, 2016). However, we need to acknowledge that firstly, most babies are not *exclusively* breastfed, especially beyond the first 6-8 weeks (Infant Feeding Survey, 2010). Secondly, even optimally breastfed babies do sometimes become unwell. Most of the time, children are admitted to hospital for a relatively short duration (Neill et al, 2018), indeed one retrospective study found that the average length of stay for under-fives is 1.8 days (Heys et al, 2017). They may not even be admitted, but just assessed in the Emergency Department or reviewed on a Rapid Assessment Unit and yet, this might be enough time to damage their breastfeeding journey. Admissions to the paediatric unit do not have to be long in duration to have a significant negative impact on breastfeeding duration and exclusivity.

Any child who is unwell or unstable enough with an acute illness will be admitted to the children's ward, High Dependency Unit (HDU) or Paediatric Intensive Care Unit (PICU). This may be to receive oxygen therapy, non-invasive breathing support, IV fluids, antibiotics, and observation – often a combination of several of these. Other children may need more invasive support, such as organ support and mechanical ventilation. An acute illness is short in duration, perhaps just days or a few weeks, but that does not mean it is not traumatic, distressing or severe. Furthermore, some acute infections can have long term consequences – for example, hypoxia, intracranial swelling or haemorrhage can lead to brain damage.

Archie was an 8-week-old baby who was admitted with sepsis. He spent a week on the ward, and during that time his mother was told to only feed him every four hours. There is rarely any clinical rationale for four-hourly feeding and this mother knew that. She was well-informed and committed to breastfeeding. She knew that if her baby was not feeding well, she needed to protect her supply. The ward did not provide a pump, and so this mother was forced to hand express and discard her milk over the sink next to her baby's cot, in an open ward with very little privacy in order to maintain her supply.

One study that I have previously referred to explored the impact of admission to hospital with an acute illness and is, to my knowledge, the only paper exploring the impact of an acute illness on breastfeeding outcome (Heilbronner et al, 2017). This was a cross sectional study in France, exploring the experiences of 84 breastfeeding mother-baby pairs. All the infants in this study were admitted with bronchiolitis. Some of the infants were admitted to PICU, and they received oxygen therapy, CPAP or were ventilated.

The study found that being admitted to hospital was strongly associated with reduction or cessation of breastfeeding, and this finding was unrelated to severity of illness or length of stay. In fact, more than half the mothers in this study had altered breastfeeding status as a direct result of the admission – either cessation or reduced exclusivity. Cessation of breastfeeding was slightly more likely with younger infants. The most common reason cited by mothers in the study for reduction or cessation of breastfeeding was medical advice.

How is breastfeeding negatively impacted?

So, if the severity or duration of illness is not a major factor in the modification of breastfeeding, what is? Well, I wonder how many of you recognize some of these common scenarios. These are all either phrases I have heard myself, or phrases that mothers have told me were said to them:

- Fluid charts (writing down the number of minutes without an accurate feed assessment).
- Calculated volumes by infant weight per feed.
- Equating a long feed with a large volume and vice versa.

- "Only feed for 10 minutes."
- "They need to be on the breast for 30 minutes."
- "Your baby will get too tired breastfeeding."
- "Your baby won't be able to."
- "Why don't you express to see how much milk you're making?"
- "Your baby's health is more important."
- "Your baby is still hungry because they'll take a bottle."

Fluid balance *is* important, but when it comes to breastfeeding, sometimes staff appear totally flummoxed about what to write down when a baby breastfeeds. They feel the need to objectify the feed somehow, so usually end up writing down things like 8 minutes left side, or 11 minutes right side. This *does not mean anything at all* without an assessment of effective milk transfer. It's also common for mothers to feel stressed and overwhelmed when they are told they need to provide a certain specific volume of milk every three hours. Usually this is based on the infant's weight but can be wholly unrealistic in the early days of lactation, and it often derails parental confidence. It is also, as previously mentioned, not physiologically normal with breastfed infants. The amount of milk produced remains fairly consistent between one to six months. This means that if an infant is prescribed 150ml/kg, this will happen to work out at around 750ml in 24 hours for a 5kg infant. This may be perfectly achievable, but if the infant is 8kg, this equates to 1200ml in 24 hours and may be wholly unrealistic on a practical level. But it also belies the way that breastfeeding works - remember that human milk is adaptive and dynamic, constantly changing to meet the needs of the child. The micro and macronutrient levels alter across the day, according to the frequency of feeding, and due to signalling from the child.

Closely related to these are the assumptions that a long feed means a large volume of milk, and vice versa – but since babies do not all drink in the same way, and because flow rates from the breast are not constant, this is not true, and can either discourage, or falsely reassure.

Another common idea that I run into a lot is that babies will get tired from breastfeeding. This notion needs some unpacking because, as I have already said, oral feeding *does* cause a degree of physiological stress, but there is no evidence that breastfeeding is *more* tiring than bottle feeding. In fact, the opposite is true, and so if an infant is too unstable to breastfeed, they are arguably too unstable to orally feed with any method. There is also often an assumption about whether babies can breastfeed based on their diagnosis. This is not a fair speculation, as all babies respond differently. We should make individual assessments of feeding competence, rather than write babies off on the basis of their diagnosis, or assume that they are too sick to feed.

Then there are the more overtly unhelpful and passive aggressive comments. I have known many mothers who were asked *'have you finished yet?'*, or *'are they still feeding?'*, *'Are they actually feeding, or just using you as a dummy?'*. These are hurtful and dismissive of the many other beneficial aspects of breastfeeding; they are demeaning and unsupportive.

I've also sadly heard some inappropriate suggestions, such as using the volumes expressed with a pump as a gauge for how much milk a mother is making. Pumps are not perfect substitutes for effectively feeding babies, and a mother under pressure does not always find it easy to pump, especially when people are piling on pressure to produce certain volumes every time. It's a recipe for a breastfeeding breakdown.

Then there are the emotive and guilt-inducing statements that are often very dichotomous. I've heard these especially from parents of critically sick children – statements like *'your baby's health is more important'*, or *'your baby is still hungry'*. No loving parent would ever say that breastfeeding was more important than their baby's life, and yet that is what these statements inadvertently imply. It implies that breastfeeding, or wanting to continue to breastfeed is inherently selfish, or mainly for the mother's benefit. It devalues breastfeeding as a part of mothering and parenting, and the importance of human milk for children.

And all this is before we get to the equipment – no pumps in sight, or the reluctance to put expressed milk in the same fridge as food, and so on.

Supporting breastfeeding in the paediatric setting

So, how do we get around the barriers and make breastfeeding support happen in paediatrics? I think there are six steps we can consider when a breastfed child is admitted to the paediatric ward or PICU:

1. We can ask about infant feeding goals. I don't just mean how the child is being fed in a mechanical sense – 'breast or bottle', as if the only difference is the milk delivery vessel. But really digging down into this. What does the mother want? When they first thought about breastfeeding, did they have any goals in mind? Has anything changed? How can their goals be communicated to the rest of the healthcare team? Reassuring the mother that their goals remain important in spite of, and perhaps because of, their child's illness.

2. The paediatric infant feeding team is notified and easily accessible. A designated infant feeding team located on the paediatric floor, experienced in breastfeeding issues in older babies and toddlers, and specifically trained to support sick children. This important team would be able to advocate for the family as well as liaising with and collaborating with the medical team, so that the mother can just get on with caring and feeding their child, and not have to defend their right to breastfeed.

3. Peer supporters available on the phone at any time of the day or night, who are aware that sometimes adaptations are needed for a sick infant or child.

4. Equipment made available and treated as a priority. This means that the staff aren't cluelessly ringing round other departments trying to borrow equipment from the NICU or postnatal ward, where it is probably in short supply anyway. No more mothers becoming uncomfortably engorged in the ED because nobody has thought about whether to offer the mother a pump. Equipment would be designated to the paediatric department, and its provision for mothers offered proactively, without a frustrating and sometimes debilitating delay.

5. Assess individual lactation needs. This means that we do not assume that a baby with Down syndrome will have low tone

and trouble with milk transfer. We do not write off a baby with a heart defect, or neuroblastoma, assuming that they will need formula. We start with the assumption that adaptations may be required, but breastfeeding goals can still be met, with creativity and individualization. We also do not forget that while breastfeeding problems may be complex, and condition-specific, mothers may also have the common or garden varieties of breastfeeding issues. Mastitis, blocked ducts, blebs and hyperlactation still happen in mothers of medically complex children. Staff need to be equipped to either support a range of challenges, or refer to specialist lactation professionals.

6. Co-create a plan with the family, taking their wishes, priorities, goals and specific challenges and strengths into account. The plan will be communicated to the wider healthcare team, valued and upheld.

The evidence I've found so far suggests that a blueprint for effective paediatric lactation provision might look something like this: The child's condition is obviously treated or managed effectively, and the family is involved in all decision making. The lactation needs of the family are identified and those are incorporated into the healthcare plan. The staff on the unit are willing to be flexible and offer creative solutions to enable and facilitate breastfeeding or the provision of human milk. Breastfeeding is valued as part of the child and family's care, including the management of any challenges, whether common, or highly specific to the child's condition. There is adequate provision and explanation of how to use equipment such as pumps, so that the comfort and wellbeing of the mother as well as the need for milk of the infant can be prioritised.

Finally, in all areas of care, there is a multidisciplinary approach to meet the needs of the family in a holistic way. See Chapter 8 for my multi-disciplinary decision-making framework for breastfed children on the paediatric ward which aims to guide your next steps and can be used alongside a feeding assessment.

Feeding assessments

You may need some more specific tips if you want to start out with making feeding assessments part of the admission process. Obviously, you will be guided by the child's age, as well as the mother's feeding goals and their past and current feeding history. Then consider, in light of the child's actual or working diagnosis, what interventions may interfere with or interrupt breastfeeding responsively. Ask the family if there are any barriers interrupting the maintenance of feeding – for example, do they have another breastfed child at home, or are they particularly stressed about something.

Then get practical – what does this family need in order to be able to continue breastfeeding? Do they need equipment, a bigger bed, some emotional support? If the child has a clinical need for supplementation, how can this be done to minimise the disruption to feeding – is supplementing with the mother's own milk a possibility, could donor milk be used? Could the breast milk be fortified to add calories without adding volume? How can the infant continue to be comforted even if they cannot directly feed – consider interventions such as non-nutritive suckling on a well-drained breast, as well as skin to skin, bedsharing, or wearing the child in a sling or carrier.

Consider how to reassure and encourage mothers who are unable to breastfeed in the way that they would wish. It can feel very demoralising to hear that breastfeeding or breast milk is inappropriate for a child, no matter how legitimate the clinical rationale. Many mothers have explained that they can be grateful that their child is safely fed, but still mourn the loss of the feeding experience that they hoped for (Brown, 2019). Having compassionate conversations with mothers, listening to their story, and reassuring them of the value of breast milk for the bigger picture of their child's health is important. One mother I spoke to was distressed at needing to use high calorie formula to PEG feed her child. She rationalised the situation in her mind by considering that she was *inclusively* breastfeeding, rather than *exclusively* breastfeeding. This mindset shift helped her to compartmentalise the high calorie formula as a medical treatment.

And finally, how can this infant be returned to the breast as soon as possible? Will any adaptation be needed, and how can we prepare in advance so there is no delay in returning the child to their usual feeding experience? In many paediatric wards, the estimated discharge date is recorded. Why can't we have the same approach to feeding? Estimated return to breast date? I'm sure someone could think of something catchier!

Different feeding assessment tools

There are a variety of feeding assessment tools that have been developed over many years. The Infant Breastfeeding Assessment Tool - IBFAT (Matthews, 1988), the LATCH Tool (Jensen et al, 1994), the Mother Baby Assessment Tool - MBA (Mulford, 1992), the Preterm Newborn Breastfeeding Behaviour Scale - PIBBS (Nyqvist and Ewald, 1999) and the Neonatal Oral-Motor Assessment Scale - NOMAS (Palmer et al, 1993).

There is not a consensus on which one is the most valid, reliable or effective at either predicting or identifying problems. In all likelihood, different tools probably work better for different children and practitioners also develop preferences which often helps them get more out of an assessment. In addition to the feeding assessment tools I've mentioned, there are also tongue tie assessment tools. Some of the feeding assessment and tongue tie tools require training to administer.

Of all the tools I have seen, the Feeding Flock tools developed by Britt Pados (Pados et al, 2017) in Canada seem to be the most relevant to the paediatric population where children may have complex medical needs. This is a great set of fairly new feeding assessment tools that have shown promise in studies of the older paediatric population, with tools available for infants older than and younger than seven months, for breastfed as well as bottle fed infants and children who are eating solids.

There are numbers to score, and it is intended to be used to guide clinical decision making and discussion about next steps. Areas of challenge may involve both mother and child – for example if there are no audible swallows and the child is otherwise showing clear signs of readiness to feed and suckles actively, then the tool may guide professionals to explore maternal causes, such as inhibited milk ejection reflex, and address that as a priority.

The tool also identifies behaviours that indicate a child may need more support or may have an underlying reason for their behaviour during feeding, such as gurgling noises, choking and desaturation. A baby exhibiting these behaviours should trigger some further assessment. Unlike other tools, this one is intended to be family-centred, respecting both the parent's opinion as well as their experience of feeding.

You can download these tools from the Feeding Flock website for free: www.feedingflock.com

What to *do* with an assessment?

In terms of what to do next, using a tool should guide a practitioner to know how best to respond. It should not be the last thing someone does, unless the infant is absolutely ready to feed. Otherwise, the tools should be used as a guide, to both highlight strengths and plan the next steps based on the identified challenges.

If a child is struggling, it is always worth reviewing the basics. Could the positioning be improved? Could the mother be guided to support their child in a different way to make it easier for them? Then you may need to consider underlying causes and work out whether these are maternal in origin – such as low milk supply or inhibited milk ejection reflex, or infant related in origin – such as respiratory distress, disorganised suckle, low tone, tongue tie, or fatigue. These children may need additional support, more time, or a flexible approach to feeding.

Remember that it's not all or nothing – if we consider readiness to feed as a beginning, rather than the end point of entirely independent baby led, cue based responsive feeding, this allows some flexibility around allowing the baby to feed directly when they are stable or ready, and backing off when they show signs that they are not ready. Babies have good and difficult days, better, and then more difficult moments, and we should not presume that readiness to feed is a linear trajectory.

Finally, any tool should guide a practitioner and parent to think of creative solutions. There may not actually *be* a solution every time, but we should consider whether there is a workaround that might help the baby to feed more effectively.

I also often reassure professionals that we may be in uncharted territory when it comes to how best to feed medically complex infants and children. There may not be a best practice guideline, or conventional wisdom on how to approach a particular situation.

Sometimes we have to accept that trial and error, using our clinical judgement, and involving other more experienced colleagues is what is required. If we do this, we should not be afraid to be honest with the family and acknowledge that nobody is certain. Try out a technique or approach, and review it at the next feed, or whenever it is clinically appropriate.

To improve the experiences of medically complex children and their families, we need to recognize that practical and psychological support is often needed for mothers, partners and indeed the child and siblings as well, if they are old enough. We need to value the role of breastfeeding and the provision of human milk as medicine for a sick child. We need to extend the family centred care ethos into lactation care in the paediatric setting and provide individualised lactation support according to need. We should provide training and mentorship to lactation professionals who are supporting sick and complex children, and equally, we should provide training to healthcare professionals about lactation and the role of human milk in the care of children.

Finally, we need to ensure adequate provision of equipment and resources and train all staff who may need to use or promote them in how to use them.

Test yourself:

1. Breastfeeding cessation is related to the severity of infant illness.
   a. True/False.
2. Feeding assessments should consider which aspects of lactation?
   a. Parental feeding goals.
   b. Infant age.
   c. What clinical procedures may interfere with feeding?
   d. All the above.
3. Which of the following is supportive of breastfeeding?
   a. Asking how long a baby has been feeding.
   b. Telling a mother that they need to produce 90ml every 3 hours.
   c. Asking them how they feel their feeding is going.
   d. Suggesting that bottle feeding might be easier for them.
4. How should you use a feeding assessment tool?
   a. To highlight strengths and challenges.
   b. To reassure a mother that their child is ready to try feeding.
   c. To diagnose problems.
   d. All except c.

Chapter 6

Parent stories and portraits of bravery

There is often nothing more powerful than the story of someone who has experienced adversity. Evidence and data are really important, but so is conveying the lived experience of the mothers (and often fathers too) who are affected by these issues.

For as long as I have been captivated by this topic, I have been listening to the stories of families. You know my story already of course, but there is enormous value in hearing from a range of parents with children of different ages, persevering through different conditions, and having a variety of positive and negative experiences. Some were acutely unwell for a short time, others battled on for many months.

Alongside my PhD I have, with several members of the Breastfeeding the Brave group, been trying different strategies to educate and raise awareness of the challenges facing parents of sick children. So far, I have created a YouTube video featuring many of our collected stories, as well as raising awareness via social media. This book incorporates a project utilising art. I asked for parents who wanted to share their story to come forward and I'm grateful for the hundreds of shares this post received on social media.

I was blown away by the response I had from mothers around the world who wanted to share their story with me. Whilst there are many examples of excellent practice, for some of the mothers this was the first time someone had taken notice of their struggle and acknowledged the hard work, frustration and difficulty of breastfeeding through medical complexity in the paediatric setting.

Hundreds of mothers came forward, eager to celebrate their child's bravery, as well as their fierce determination. Leanne Pearce, an artist known for her art with purpose, chose several images with me. We wanted to showcase these amazing mothers, in the hope that professionals will understand the research by connecting with the stories through the art.

Healthcare has often been described as an art and a science, and yet art in healthcare teaching is not a commonly utilised approach though it may help practitioners become more compassionate and empathic (Darbyshire, 1994; Wikström, 2001; Zazulak et al, 2017).

Many families in the Breastfeeding the Brave group have had long, difficult and sometimes traumatic experiences and often for this reason, they are keen to tell their story. The thought that their experience may influence professional care and reduce suffering even for one other parent is often a big motivator for wanting to share.

I think that art may be an innovative way to convey the difficulties and unique experience of this population group in a way that simply sharing research literature may not (Hookway, 2022).

We hope that these incredible paintings will illustrate some of the differences and challenges in the paediatric setting. This is particularly important when it is such an under-researched area and some are simply unaware that there are many differences in this population, and the ways they should be cared for. Art and stories that depict aspects of unresearched care may increase the prevalence of care-giving behaviours such as skin to skin, holding and breastfeeding very sick children.

We chose a range of ages of children with many different conditions for the paintings, and we also tried to show real experiences in all their raw vulnerability. We actively chose to depict fathers with their children, as well as mothers, because partners are so often forgotten, and we know that the support of a partner greatly increases the likelihood of breastfeeding goals being met. I've included some stories and images of children who have sadly died because their stories are meaningful. Furthermore, breastfeeding through palliative illness and coping with bereavement is an important part of family centred infant feeding support and it would be remiss of me to leave these children and their mothers out.

How art may be used in healthcare

Some of the accompanying stories are very moving, and not all of them have a happy ending. These aspects of paediatric care are important to represent as well, and in fact, while many people are known to derive enjoyment from looking at pleasant images, it is also true that pictures which depict a sadder story are deeply impactful. It's why some people are drawn to a weepy movie or a tragic novel. These negative emotions invoke a profound response in many people, and this is also important (Menninghaus et al, 2017; Mastandrea, 2019).

Our hope is that many healthcare settings may display prints of these incredible portraits, and we hope to inspire more artwork in the paediatric setting that will inspire both other parents, as well as professionals. We hope they will start conversations, inspire discussion or prompt questions, as well as help people process difficult situations, think of creative solutions and acknowledge some of the hard parts of paediatric care in a non-threatening way. My other hope is that the art provides an inspiring sense of possibility for breastfeeding in a situation where it might otherwise feel impossible.

The artwork you will see in this chapter provides a window into the private and often unseen world of the realities of breastfeeding children through medical complexity and gives the message that breastfeeding against the odds *is* possible.

Leanne has done an absolutely incredible job of capturing the poignancy of some of these amazing parents. For every portrait you observe, there are hundreds of other stories. We are so grateful to these art-in-healthcare ambassadors for their courage to share these moments.

I hope that reading through their stories, and looking at their portraits tells a story that all the research in the world cannot hope to tell. I am indebted to these families for allowing us to bring their voice into the public domain.

To Hannah, Cara, Anna, Alice, Shurron, Laura, Gemma, Rachel – we thank you.

** Warning: these stories include experiences of serious childhood illness, resuscitation and infant death which some readers may find distressing. **

Hannah and Maisie

I have breastfed all three of my children (our youngest I am still feeding). Our middle child - Maisie - was very ill throughout her life, and sadly passed away just before she turned six months old after battling a heart condition and mitochondrial disease. Although she spent a lot of time in hospital, she was exclusively breastfed. When Maisie was seriously ill in PICU, I would pump as much as I could and it was really beneficial to have the task of pumping to make me feel useful and to distract me from how critically ill she was but I was never offered any help or advice about pumping or breastfeeding a sick child at any of the hospitals or wards.

During her first admission for her heart surgery it was so hard to see her look at me and suck on her breathing tube as she wanted to feed so badly, but couldn't as she was too ill. The day before her operation (which happened to be my birthday), the team gave me the opportunity to hold her again. It was scary, but we were so happy - her breathing and heart rate improved and oxygen saturations increased. [Pictured in Leanne's painting].

I found a real lack of understanding of breastfeeding amongst most of the health professionals. I was constantly asked during procedures whether she took a dummy or a bottle to soothe her - it seemed far more "normal" and expected than breastfeeding. Another issue I encountered was being allowed to co-sleep in a hospital bed with Maisie. On admission I'd have to constantly ask for a bed to share, which would often be met with mixed reactions - sometimes it would be easy, other times I'd have to sign a waiver which made me feel guilty.

Measuring input and output was a regular occurrence - I'd be asked to keep a written record of feeds and for how long. I understand why this is important - but the reality of recording the feeding of a baby who breastfeeds is impossible. She would be on and off all day, with a mixture of comfort feeds, sleepy feeds and hungry feeds.

It would really make a difference if all paediatric health professionals understood breastfeeding - especially the benefits to critically ill children, so they could help to support them. It would also be really beneficial for hospitals to understand that co-sleeping and breastfeeding often go hand-in-hand, and similarly offer incredible physical and mental health benefits for both parents and children, especially in stressful situations. It would be wonderful if lactation specialists could be on hand to offer information in every paediatric setting. I was lucky that Maisie was my second child and that I had lots of experience and confidence in breastfeeding already - but without this, I think I would have really struggled to breastfeed her at such a difficult time.

In the end, although we were aware Maisie wouldn't have a very long life, she passed away quite suddenly during a routine hospital visit. I continued to pump as she suffered a cardiac arrest, in the hope that she would be able to recover - but sadly, after a long fight, she passed away. When I picked her up after she died, she hadn't fed for over six hours, and my first instinct was to put her to my breast - it seemed so strange for her not to feed. I considered continuing to pump to donate my milk - but I found the whole thing too sad, as my milk was meant for Maisie, not another baby. I wasn't offered anything to dry my milk up, and no-one offered any advice - but a friend gave me that support instead.

One of the things I desperately wanted to do was to breastfeed a baby again - and I was incredibly fortunate to be able to do that with our rainbow baby just over two years later, Maisie's baby brother, Theo.

Breastfeeding is the most wonderful, miraculous and magical thing, and I feel truly honoured to have been able to breastfeed all three of my children. For Maisie in particular it offered her the most incredible comfort through awful pain, and the best nutrition we could ask for to keep her as well as possible. Getting the right balance between using the knowledge and experience of both parents and medical staff to make decisions can be really tough - but I think there is still huge room for improvement in paediatric care.

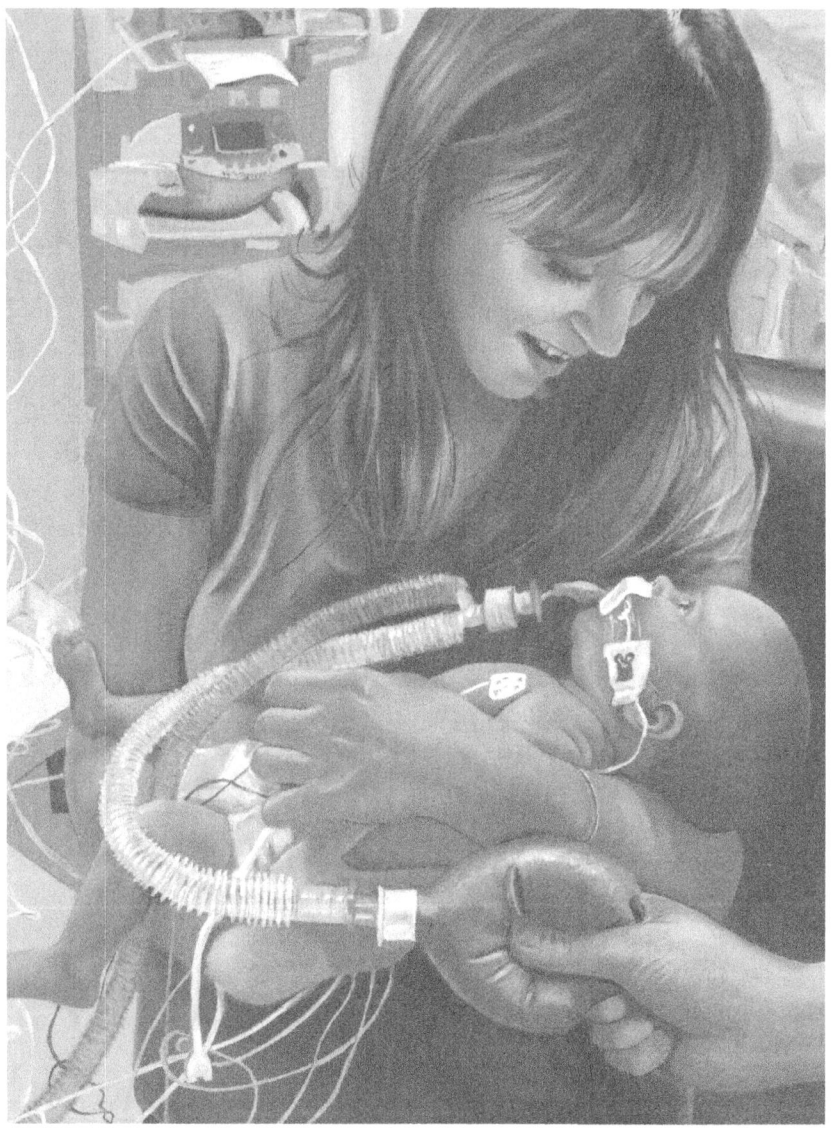

Hannah and Maisie

Cara, Jayke and Maya

My son Jayke was diagnosed with Acute Lymphoblastic Leukaemia when he was four and a half years old, I was 8 weeks postpartum and exclusively breastfeeding my newborn daughter Maya. Maya was allowed to stay on the ward with us because we were breastfeeding, the nurses were very supportive of this. After a short while, Jayke needed a feeding tube as the chemotherapy took his appetite. I started expressing milk to give through his tube. The dietitian involved with his care advised me not to, that it would provide no benefit to him. I knew this to be untrue and continued anyway.

We were inpatients for months at a time and our treatment hospital was an hour from home. With Jayke's health too unstable for us to leave when we faced breastfeeding struggles it was impossible to receive support. I attended the hospital run breastfeeding support group based in the maternity wing of the hospital, however the staff turned me away saying that Maya was too old and we didn't have a local residence. The nearest volunteer run group was too far from the hospital to travel to, it was a very isolated and overwhelming experience trying to find the right support.

Four months after Jayke's diagnosis we discovered a lump on Maya's chest and she was quickly diagnosed with Fibromatosis, a tumour on her chest wall. We were still exclusively breastfeeding at this time which she found very comforting through her procedures, however we were given incorrect and inconsistent guidance regarding breast milk while fasting for surgical procedures under anaesthetic. We reached out to lactation consultants privately who were able to give us the right information and despite resistance and hesitation from hospital staff they have let us lead the way with breastfeeding over the years, trusting that what I am saying is true because they have little information.

I have continued to breastfeed through the children's medical journey for the past three years. Unfortunately this has been entirely without professional support as it just doesn't seem to be available at present.

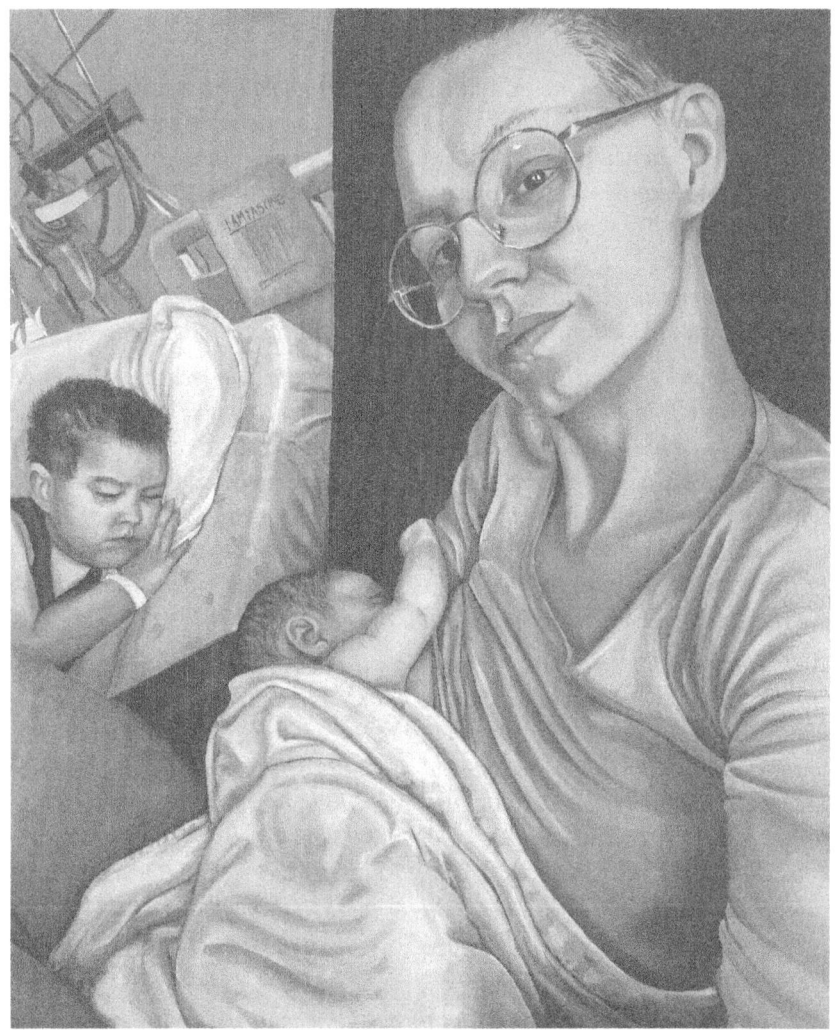

Cara, Jayke and Maya

Anna

Both our kids were born prematurely so hospitals and pumping were familiar. When our younger son was diagnosed with dilated cardiomyopathy and Hirschsprung's disease at 14 weeks and fighting for his life in PICU at least I had some knowledge of what to do. But having a breastfed baby on paediatric wards was totally different to NICU. Thank god I already knew how to use the hospital pump and what volumes to aim for. Someone did talk me through it quickly on the PICU but it was soon after they told me the severity of my son's condition and nothing was going in.

He was ventilated and nil by mouth, but I knew I needed to pump to keep up supply and avoid mastitis. The parents' accommodation for PICU was off-site and no spare pumps meant regularly heading back up to PICU - even at 3am. It gave me a chance to check on my son but it was exhausting.

When they told us they had done everything they could I remember staring at the pump and nothing coming out. I had always had good milk volumes so this was catastrophic to me.

No one checked how pumping was going and nobody told me what to do when this happened. Of course when the worst had passed my milk came back in abundance. But at that moment I was in despair. This happened during the first covid lockdown and my partner wasn't allowed to be with me. Trying to hold together all the medical information, consistently pumping, and the emotions of being told our kid might not survive, doing all this alone, I will never ever get over.

If I hadn't successfully breastfed my older child and pumped before, I think I may not have been able to continue. But I knew that if we came out of this I needed to be able to breastfeed. Though my production on PICU was abysmal, I had a freezer stash from NICU so when he was allowed to have NG feeds he received my milk. There was no way I could have kept up otherwise. The trauma was showing in my supply.

Eventually we moved to the cardiac HDU. They were very supportive of breastfeeding even though they measured fluid input and output. My pet hate was nurses warming a whole bottle of breast milk! The rest then has to go in the bin. It literally fills me with rage. That admission was five weeks and his surgery for Hirschsprungs was ten days. The whole time, apart from the hours they thought he wouldn't make it, my partner wasn't allowed to be in the hospital or the parents' accommodation. PICU was an hour away from our home and my older son (who was also still breastfeeding) and that family separation was unbearable.

We rented a flat nearby so when I came off the ward we could be together. The times I got to feed my older son were so important to me as time with him was scarce. Eventually, a few days before we came home my partner was allowed on the ward. This picture is the moment he got to hold his son again after a 5 week fight for his life.

Once we were home, breastfeeding went back to normal. However, my son was on diuretics and nobody talked to us about fluid levels. I was anxious about vomiting as it was a big trigger for me from before he was diagnosed. So I wouldn't let him feed too much just in case. Consequently he got quite dehydrated and ended up with an acute kidney injury. I wish there had been better support for breastfeeding and how to ensure he was getting enough fluid, but it was like no one had thought of it. Thankfully once off his diuretic his kidneys recovered though he will be under the renal team for life.

Breastfeeding has always been important to me. I wish I could carry my kids to term but I will always be somewhat grateful for the time I spent in the NICU which set me up for when my younger son was desperately ill. Without that pumping knowledge and freezer stash I don't think we could have come through with our breastfeeding relationship intact.

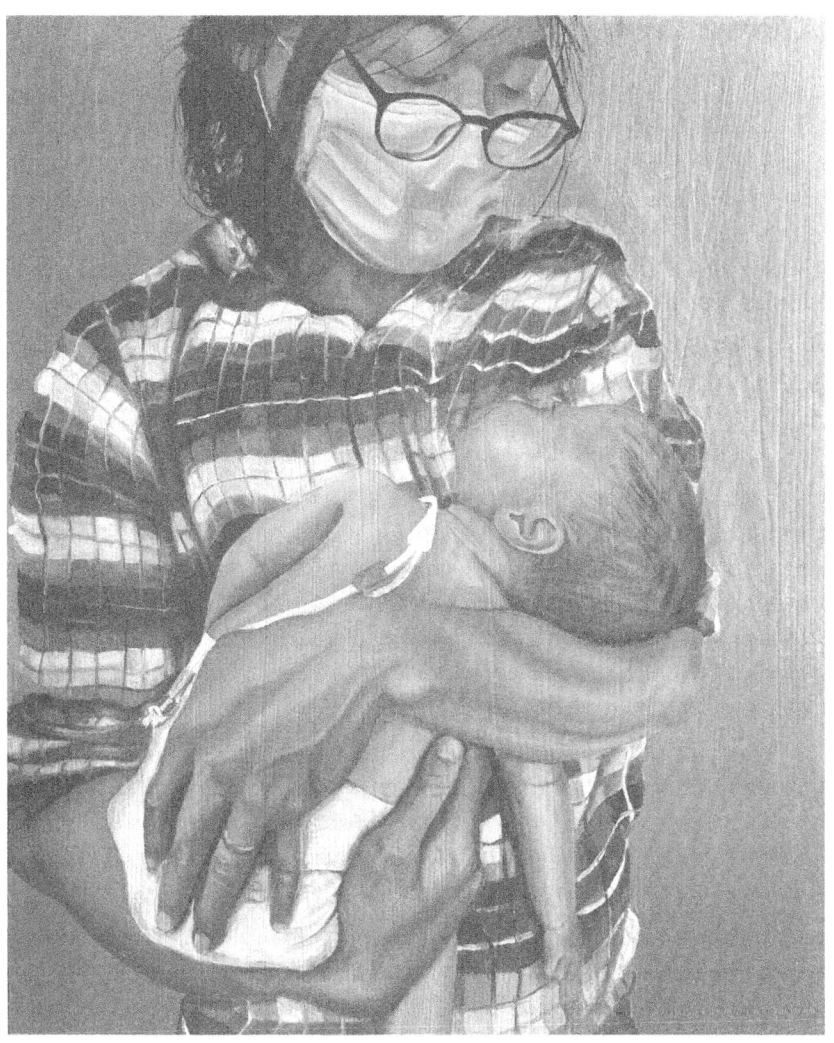

Anna and Will

Alice and Ash

My husband and I tried for years to have a baby and were overjoyed when our first IVF cycle was successful. The pregnancy was mostly uneventful so it was quite a surprise when at 30 weeks I went into spontaneous labour in front of my Year 6 Class! My teaching assistant rushed me to hospital and a few days later Ash was born – weighing just 3lbs. Little by little, Ash was weaned off life support until two months later we were finally given the all clear to take him home.

As July gave way to August, our days settled into a comforting, happy rhythm until one evening our lives were turned upside down. Ash suddenly refused to breastfeed and a familiar blue tinge returned to his skin. I recognised the signs immediately and we rushed him to A&E.

The nurse there treated me like a neurotic mother and (with an infuriatingly patronising tone) repeatedly reassured me that he was fine and to take him home. Thank god I stood my ground and forced them to take me seriously. His oxygen levels were so low that night that he had to be put into a coma, onto a ventilator and rushed to Great Ormond Street where he was diagnosed with RSV. If I had gone home when I was asked to, I dread to think what may have happened.

Early on in the coma, his vitals dipped dangerously low and he required two minutes of CPR and a shot of adrenaline to bring him back to us. He spent 7 long weeks fighting for his life and I'm not sure we will ever fully recover from the trauma of nearly losing him so many times and having to witness him experiencing so much pain and fear.

Because Ash was so unwell, I was unable to hold him. Parents are not allowed to sleep in Intensive Care (not even a little nap sat up in the chair by his bed) so we were forced to leave his bedside for agonising stretches of time. The hardest part for me was not being able to breastfeed. I desperately missed that connection and sitting alone in a hospital milk room listening to the rhythmic sound of the pump whilst scrolling through photos of him, made me incredibly sad. This sadness was further amplified when we were eventually moved from PICU to a children's ward where access to pumping facilities was less straightforward.

The pumping rooms were clinical and depressing and always locked so I'd have to go through the awkwardness of finding a nurse to unlock it, then requesting bottles, sterilising, pumping and then struggling again to find a nurse to put the expressed milk in a fridge for me (we had no access to fridges). It was really draining, I hated being away from Ash's bedside and I was constantly missing pumping times when nurses were unavailable. This reduced my supply and left me feeling frustrated and uncomfortable.

As a breastfeeding mother, I received food vouchers but they were useless as I was unable to get to the cafeteria to spend them. On the few occasions that I did attempt to buy a meal I returned to his ward room to find his alarms blaring, his eyes red with tears and no nurses to be seen either in his room or in the adjoining corridor. When this happened for the third time, I refused to leave his bedside again. The nurses were fantastic and I'm so grateful to them but there just weren't enough of them – they worked so hard. I survived on toast and cereal from the family room and meals that my husband brought in for me. Without that I'm not sure I would have been able to supply any milk at all!

The first breastfeed after he came around from the coma was an incredibly emotion'l experience. Re-establishing a connection after such a long separation, allowed us to not only bond but I was also now able to provide pain relief and comfort during painful procedures and blood transfusions (in the painting I'm feeding him during a transfusion).

Ash spent a total of 4 months in hospital during his first year of life. We recently celebrated his first birthday and he is a gentle natured, hilarious, happy little boy. We are so grateful every day that he is here with us.

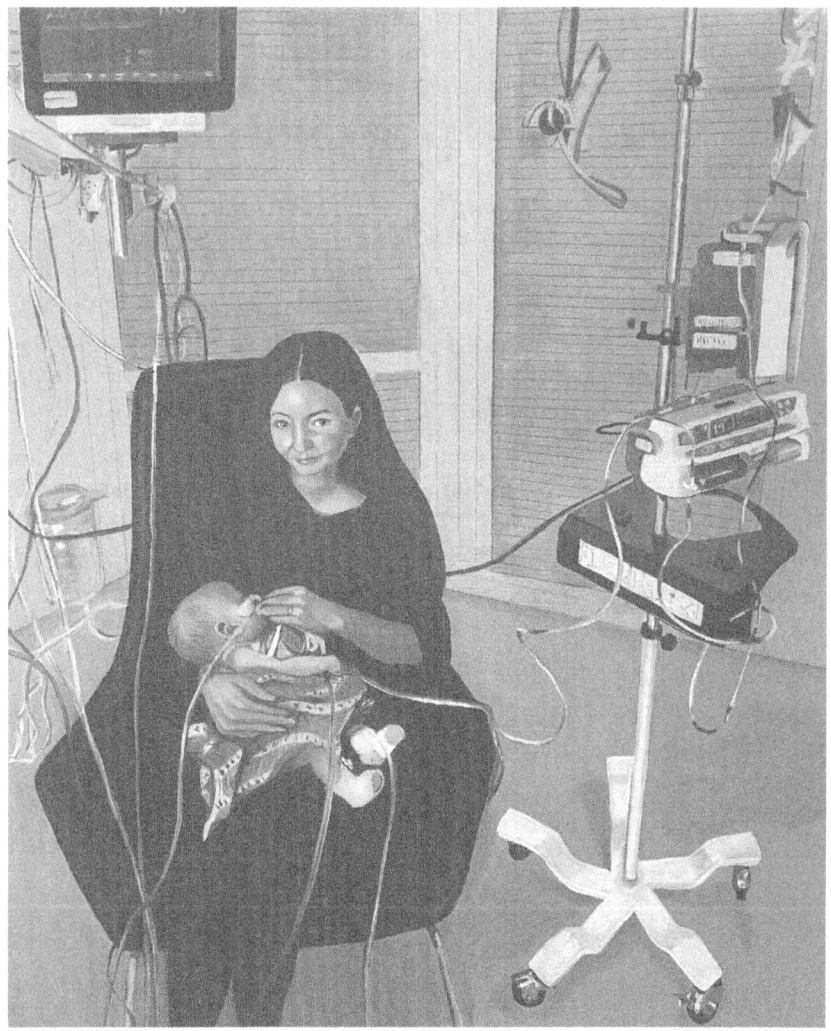

Alice and Ash

Shurron and K

After a perfectly straightforward pregnancy full of optimism, my beautiful son K was born critically ill. He was on life support in the neonatal unit for three weeks. Those three weeks were physically and emotionally battering. The birth was traumatic, I had complications after my spinal block (dural puncture) and I was separated from my son. As I was separated from him, I would smell his babygrows as I pumped every three hours, trying to get as much of my milk for him. It felt like I was living someone else's life. Like it was a terrible dream.

Pumping was tough. And my supply was low. I remember pumping 15ml and as I brought my milk into the NICU, a nurse saying to me 'is that all you have? You need to relax or your milk won't let down'. I was in the midst of trauma, doing everything I could not to fall apart. And those comments felt like a knife in my chest.

K pulled through (the first of many battles he would overcome) and I worked hard with breastfeeding specialists to increase my supply, and help K learn to feed, over the following weeks (finger feeding, supplementary lactation system, cup feeding, power-pumping – I did it all). I came close to ending my breastfeeding journey many times. But a deep, previously untapped, inner-strength of mine, emerged from the depths of my soul. It kept me going. I knew my breast milk would give K, who had so much going against him health-wise, a fighting chance at getting stronger and create the building blocks to a healthier tomorrow.

A few weeks later, and I had finally made substantial progress with my supply. But unexpectedly in the early hours of a Saturday morning, K had seizures and ended up in paediatric intensive care and on life support again. We plunged back into terror, uncertainty, a world where my son belonged to the medics and I felt my motherly instincts evaporating. That three week stay in hospital led to a life-changing diagnosis for K. He was diagnosed with a neurological condition, which had (what felt like) a very bleak outlook for K. He was diagnosed with an unsafe swallow (when bottle-feeding), and subsequently had a feeding tube inserted, so he could have milk straight into his tummy.

Breast-feeding K in hospital was important for bonding and for K to feel closeness and security. We were observed breastfeeding by so many professionals which felt medicalised and unnatural. But those moments also felt like ours. To connect and be together. They were healing to me, through a very traumatic time.

Coming home from the hospital my body felt broken. And my spirit wasn't far off. After two months of pumping every three hours, I couldn't continue on top of all the medical care we now had to give him. That's when I reached out to the Hearts Milk Bank and K was given donor human milk. With the pressure taken off me to pump, I could just focus on his medical care and trying to re-establish breastfeeding.

Within a few months, K and I had re-established breastfeeding. This meant we could bond, and I started to stitch back together the wounds that I felt tore me apart in those early days. It meant I could give him the perfect tailor-made food and antibodies that he needed on-demand. It meant he could use his mouth to feed (rather than being fed through a tube) and learn skills that I believe set him up for success with feeding and will help him with his speech. Breast milk – and those early days of donor milk supplementation – meant the world to my son, to me and to my family.

I breastfed K until he was two, when I fell pregnant with his little sister. His little sister is now two and a half, and I am still breastfeeding her. I even managed to donate milk back to the Hearts Milk Bank this time round – which felt like a really fitting way to bring my breastfeeding journey back full-circle. Breastfeeding is, hands-down, the most difficult thing I have ever done, the achievement I am proudest of. It almost broke me, but instead, revealed a strength within me that I never knew existed.

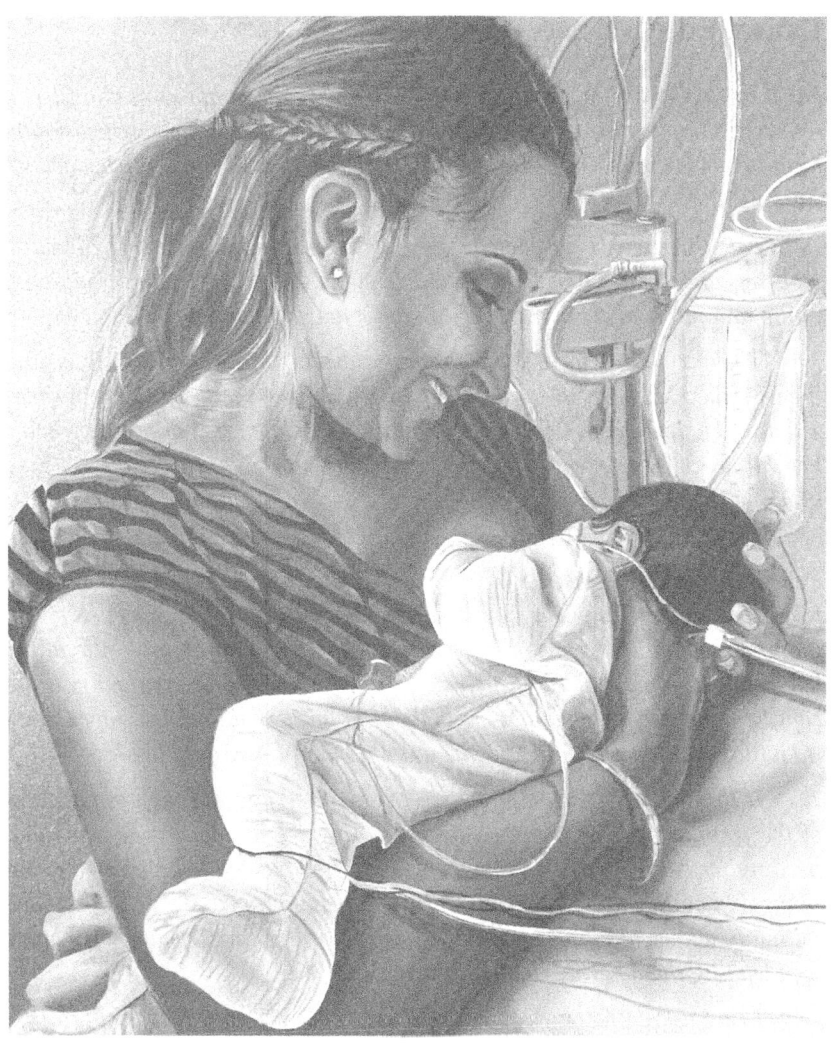

Shurron and K

Laura, Edward and Jacob

My 4 week old baby Jacob stopped breathing at home in my arms and turned blue and floppy so ended up in the HDU. During that time I turned to my local breastfeeding consultant for advice rather than the paediatricians and nursing staff.

After his apnoea episode my son was nil by mouth for the first 24 hours. Nobody said a word to me about what to do next, so I went home, found my pump and pumped every 90 mins to mimic his behaviour.

The next day he was given a feeding tube and I was allowed to give him breast milk. However, they calculated a set volume of milk and gave it every 2 hours. He had always fed every 90 minutes, so he cried and cried for the last 30 minutes before each feed. It was heart-breaking and I couldn't hold him due to the tubes etc.

I brought 210ml to the hospital with me from the previous 24 hours and for a 10ml tube feed the nurse heated the lot up so I was forced to throw it away. This left me in a pump for each feed situation. After exclusively pumping for my daughter a few years prior I'm no stranger to the pump however I was mortified to find that I was pumping little to no milk. I was coping alone due to covid and cried about my lack of milk. They topped him up with formula which stressed me out more and I produced less.

It took me a few days to realise that I was struggling to pump because of the trauma I'd been through of him having the apnoea in my arms and needing resuscitation. But nobody spoke to me about this. I brought my own pump and bottles to the hospital, sterilised them myself and wasn't provided with any advice at all. They would have just given him formula if I hadn't kept leaving them bottles of milk for the next feed.

I kept asking when I could breastfeed him again but they wouldn't let me as they needed to know exactly what he was eating, despite measuring output.

I'm not complaining about the care we received during our 5 night stay but I felt as though they were reluctant to support my breastfeeding as they were either unable to provide support or unprepared to lose control of how much he was eating during that time.

Edward adds:

I received a phone call to get to the hospital immediately, I knew it was something serious as I'd already been turned away due to the one parent covid policy. I ran into the room to find my tiny five-week-old being ventilated by hand and surrounded by a team of doctors. That night he was admitted to HDU and being nil by mouth meant that Laura could go home to get some sleep and pick up her breast pump.

Although the situation was horrible, it was nice to be able to stay with Jacob and be the one up all night with him for a change. The next morning Laura brought in her milk and I was allowed to syringe-feed a little for a comfort feed. The milk actually sent his heart rate up too high with excitement and we weren't allowed to do it for another few hours until it was safe.

For the next few days Jacob was fitted with a feeding tube and Laura's milk was provided that way instead. My role switched back to assisting with sterilising pump parts and looking after our older daughter. It wasn't an experience I'd wish to repeat but I was grateful for being able to play a key role in helping him feel safe and comfortable when only one parent was allowed to visit.

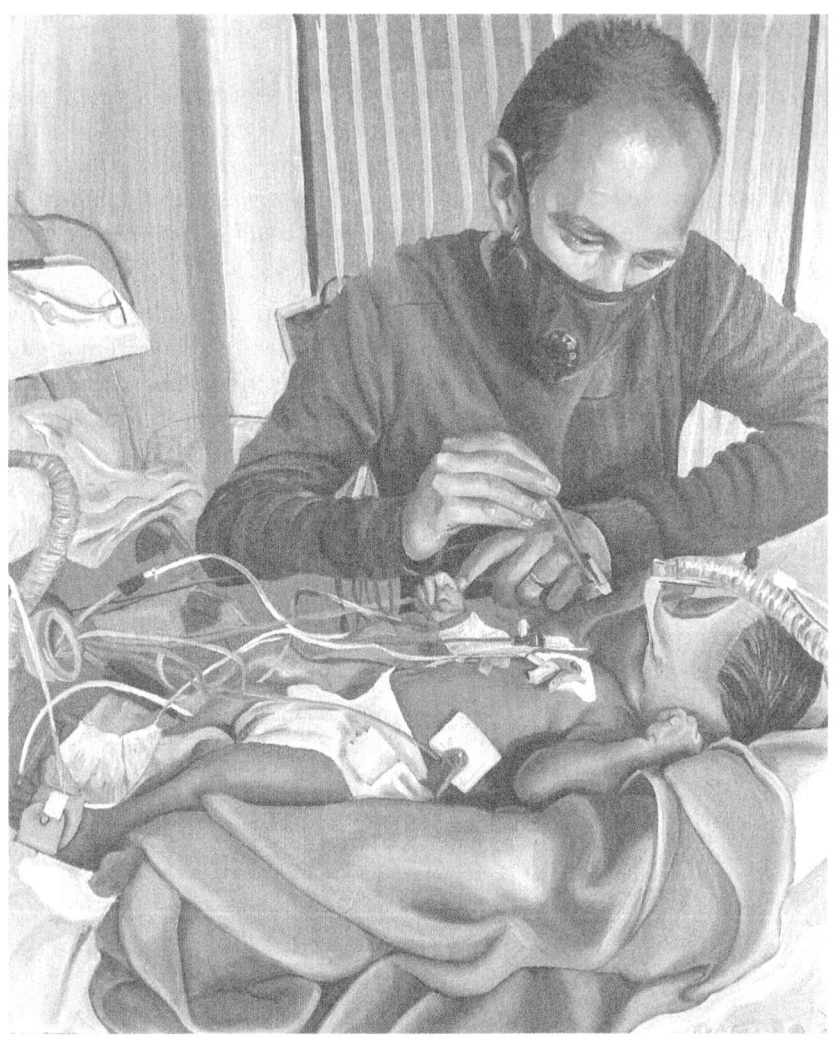

Laura, Edward and Jacob

Gemma and Benji

We had a planned home birth with my second baby, Benji, which was truly magical. However when he was 2 days old he started having seizures and stopping breathing, and we were rushed to hospital. Unfortunately due to Covid restrictions, my husband wasn't allowed into PICU until we'd all had negative covid tests, so I went up with my son alone, while he kept stopping breathing and turning blue in the lift. I was terrified.

I was given a pump and I'm so grateful this was my second baby and I'd pumped with my first, because at least I had a vague idea how to use a pump, as no-one on the ward was able to help with this. One well meaning nurse told me to pump every 3 hours during the day but only pump once overnight so I could get some sleep, but I knew that especially in the early days, overnight feeds are critical for your supply, so I pumped every 3 hours, day and night. I had to pump whilst sitting next to my tiny baby boy, intubated and covered in tubes. Luckily I had taken a "live photo" of Benji feeding just before he was taken ill, so I watched that 1.5 second clip on repeat to help. Always take photos of your baby feeding!

Benji was diagnosed with a significant subdural brain haemorrhage, the cause of which, 14 months later, is still unclear. He was initially nil by mouth but he was eventually fed my breast milk through an NG tube. This feeling that expressing milk was the only thing I could do to care for him was what kept me going in those early days. I couldn't bathe him, directly feed, cuddle him or even change his nappy, but I could make milk and that made me feel less useless. I was also supported to hold him and do skin to skin a few times (see picture), even though he had lines from every limb.

When he was strong enough to try breastfeeding it felt amazing to hold him to my breast, however he was so tired he really struggled to latch and feed. The nurses tried really hard to help and found a lovely Breastfeeding Link nurse. She wasn't able to help that much physically, however she was incredibly supportive and made a big difference to me emotionally. By this stage, despite the regular pumping, I was terribly engorged with huge lumps in my armpits and incredibly painful swollen breasts, which did not help with the latching. Eventually the nurses convinced a breastfeeding midwife from a postnatal ward to see me. She turned up with nipple shields, and Benji immediately latched and fed well. This was a bit of a double-edged sword as although he fed, it didn't improve his technique, and it took 7 months to wean him off. After that his latch was shallow which has caused months of pain, clogged ducts, bleeding nipples and vasospasm. I wish I'd had more qualified help in hospital as it could have made a big difference to our longer breastfeeding journey.

As Benji's condition improved we were moved to a standard paediatric ward, which was obviously a massive relief, but brought new challenges. My husband was no longer allowed in at all due to covid restrictions. So I had to care for my tiny baby, and I've never felt so alone and unsupported. On HDU the nurses had been weighing every nappy to check Benji was getting enough milk, but when I handed them a nappy on the paediatric ward they just dismissed me and told me to leave it on the floor by the bed. The nurses insisted on topping Benji up through his NG tube unless he fed for 15 minutes, but an 11 minute feed seemed to satiate him, and he often vomited the top ups. Given that I was pumping 70ml in 3 minutes, I felt my supply was probably such that 15 minutes was too much. I know rules can be helpful but when they're applied without thought it can be very difficult.

One of the things I found most challenging was when Benji had MRI scans. They wanted to use a technique called "feed and wrap" to avoid sedatives, which seems like a great idea (you feed the baby to sleep, then swaddle the baby to prevent them moving in the scanner). However, trying to get a baby to feed and fall asleep at a certain time is very hard! As Benji got older, it was hard to withhold feeds and sleep until an allotted time, not least because the appointments were often running an hour or so late. Twice, he woke when I transferred him to the cold MRI bed. On both occasions I was made to feel like a failure. Lots of tutting, and "popping back in" to check if I'd managed to get him back to sleep yet.

Overall I would say I'm pretty traumatised by the whole experience. Understandably my son being so close to death or severe disability was horrific, but I also feel scarred by my hospital experience. I have never felt so alone in my whole life. The NHS is under incredible strain, so I don't blame anyone for this, but I felt I was shown little empathy by most people who dealt with us. A lovely nurse snuck my husband in for an hour one evening and I will forever be in her debt.

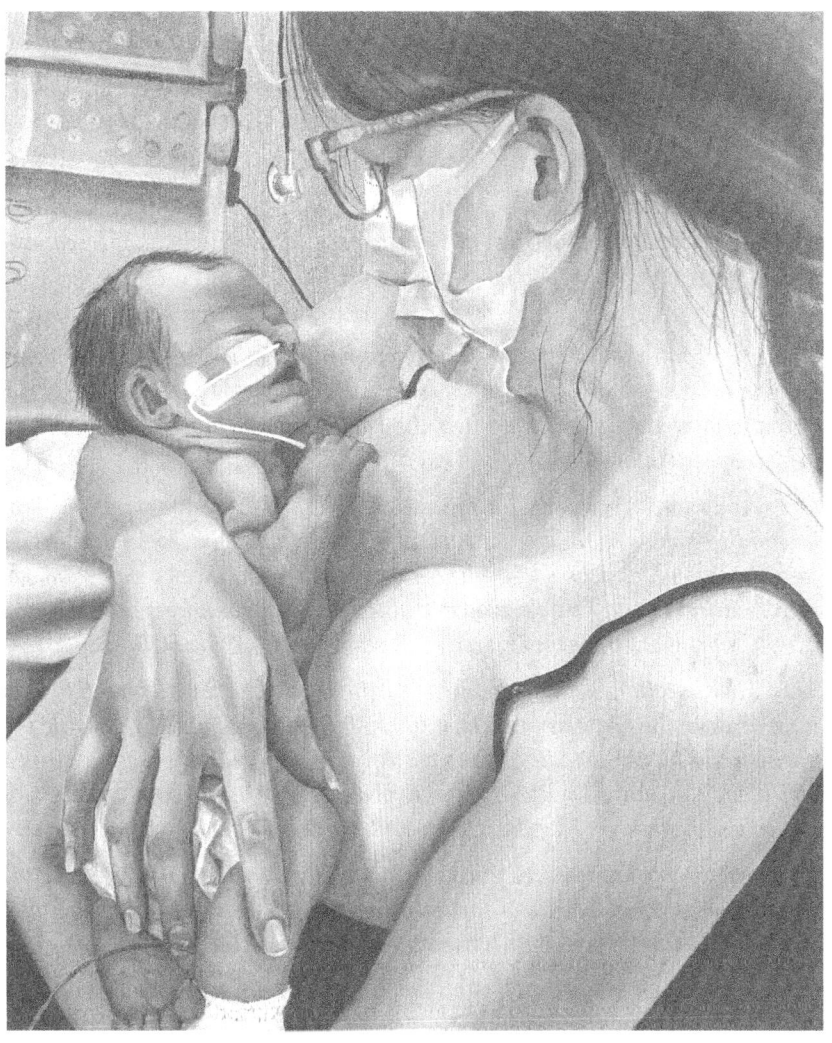

Gemma and Benji

Rachel and Etta

When I found out I was pregnant with my third child I had visions of a lovely, relaxed water birth at home. My other two labours had been straightforward so I couldn't see any reason why I couldn't have a homebirth this time around.

At 12 weeks I had the screening test. The results came back as a high chance of the baby having Down syndrome, so I was closely monitored by a consultant throughout the rest of my pregnancy.

I joined a support group on Facebook for women who have a high chance or confirmed diagnosis for Down syndrome. It was there I learned the importance of breastfeeding a baby with Down syndrome if possible. Breastfeeding can help strengthen the baby's mouth muscles, which may benefit speech later in life.

At 28 weeks my placenta began to fail, so I had weekly scans. I had to attend these alone as the country had just gone into the first lockdown. At 34 weeks it was decided to deliver the baby via C-Section. I was given 2 days of steroid injections to help develop her lungs and was talked through what to expect shortly after her birth. I was also shown around the SCBU.

The C-section went smoothly and little Etta was strong enough to stay with us until the operation was over, then she was settled in SCBU while my partner and I went to maternity to recover. Down Syndrome was confirmed by a blood test, and all initial tests were positive - she didn't seem to have any health issues that can be associated with Down syndrome.

I was shown how to harvest colostrum with syringes while I waited for the spinal block to wear off. Later that evening, my partner and I got to go visit our baby. She was tiny at 4lb1oz and perfect.

The following morning I went down to SCBU armed with my syringes to find Etta having her stomach drained. Overnight she had vomited green bile and had not yet passed meconium. The doctors thought she may have Duodenal Atresia which is a gap in the intestines. They performed an X-ray and arranged for Etta to be taken by ambulance to a bigger hospital an hour away. We followed the ambulance and Etta was taken to the NICU, while I was booked into the maternity unit at the new hospital. It was a few hours until we could see Etta and it felt like forever. She was nil by mouth, on IV antibiotics and would be having twice daily bowel washouts while they ran tests to find out what was going on, the X-ray showed she did not have Duodenal Atresia but the doctors suspected Etta had Hirschsprung's Disease.

On day 3 I was allowed to try to breastfeed. Etta latched on initially but she was weak and could not stay latched for more than a few seconds. She had an NG tube and this was used to give her my expressed milk.

Etta remained in the NICU for 3 weeks, where it was an endless cycle of expressing milk, trying to get her to latch and learning how to carry out the bowel washouts so I could perform them at home. Unfortunately I could never produce enough breast milk so Etta was mainly formula fed. She also wasn't strong enough to latch on to my breast, so I decided to try her with a bottle. She managed to take some milk from a bottle, so she was fed orally until she was too tired, then the remaining feed would go through the NG tube. Once I was signed off as competent with both bowel washouts and NG feeding, we were allowed home to wait for Etta to grow big enough for a bowel biopsy.

After 3 weeks Etta had grown strong enough to finish her feeds orally so her NG tube was removed.

A month later Etta became unwell so we rushed back to hospital. She had Enterocolitis and was put back on IV antibiotics for a week. The doctors were keen to give Etta an ileostomy, however her bowel biopsy ruled out Hirschsprung's Disease. Etta was diagnosed with bowel dysmotility and medication was prescribed.

My vision of a relaxed, natural birth and a fully breastfed baby may have gone completely out of the window, but I am thankful for the amazing people who cared for us both, and my tiny fighter who didn't let anything get in her way!

Etta will be two very soon. She is incredibly cheeky and wins the hearts of everyone around her.

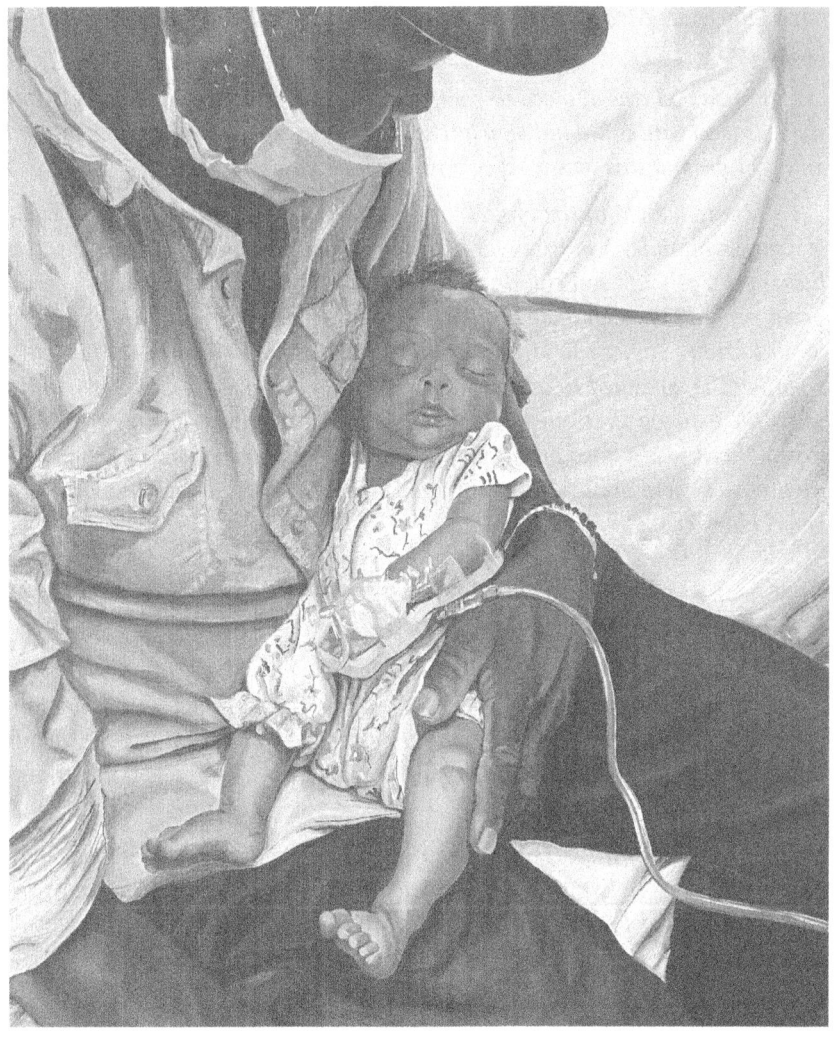

Rachel, Gladstone and Etta

Every child and family's story is unique. While I hope these stories have given you some food for thought, I encourage you to be curious and compassionate as you seek to understand the stories of those you work with. We will never truly understand the journey that a family has walked, but we can start by accepting that we will never understand. This attitude of curiosity and kindness goes a long way to helping parents feel like their experience is meaningful and important. Remember, you may have a list of patients or clients to see, but for that one family, this child is their world.

Chapter 7

Keeping the milk going

If, for any reason, babies or children are unable to feed from the breast, it is essential to keep the milk production going. Perhaps this sounds like an obvious point, but I run into so many mothers whose child hasn't been able to feed due to illness, instability, or because of the nature of their condition, and nobody has thought to tell the mother that if they don't keep removing milk, their body will downregulate milk production. This is the 'use or lose it' concept. Milk-making is a hugely high energy process, and the body is extremely efficient. If it does not need to invest energy in making milk, it won't. We cannot simply switch milk production on and off as we need it.

In real terms, if a mother does not protect her milk supply, or does not pump frequently enough, when the baby is ready to go to the breast, the milk simply won't be there – either at all, or in enough quantity to meet the baby's needs. Then the mother may either have to work really hard to get their milk supply back, or it may actually be the end of their breastfeeding journey. This may be extremely distressing for a mother who has not willingly made this choice.

Babies and children may not be able to feed directly from the breast for a vast number of reasons. You know already that even feeding under optimal conditions means a small degree of physiological stress, particularly in terms of oxygen desaturation and bradycardia. While a desaturation to 95% is fine for an uncompromised baby, if that infant's baseline oxygen saturation is 93%, then they may desaturate to below 90% during feeding. This may be an intolerable level of compromise for a baby with respiratory distress or cardiac problems.

It may be that the child is ventilated, critically unwell or unstable. Sometimes the feeding pause is due to pre-operative fasting and then a gap while the baby has surgery and recovers. Or perhaps the infant is fluid restricted and unable to drink as much as they usually do. There are many legitimate reasons to pause feeding, and so long as this is managed appropriately, there is no reason why normal feeding cannot resume once the baby is stable or their condition is managed.

But it's simply not enough to pump once or twice a day. Remember that milk production is driven by the degree of breast fullness, and influenced by milk storage capacity. There certainly may be *some* mothers who can get away with only pumping three to four times per day if their storage capacity is very large, but it would be a big gamble to assume this in advance. It's best to assume an average milk storage capacity and recommend pumping as often as their baby would usually feed.

If you are supporting an exclusively breast milk fed baby who has never been well enough to feed directly, then recommend aiming for at least 8 pumping sessions in 24 hours. These do not necessarily have to be strictly every three hours. Mothers can cluster pump at a time that suits them, and then plan to have a four or five hour gap overnight if they need to catch up on some sleep. Just make sure to educate the mother about the importance of pumping at least once in the early hours of the morning. In practice, many mothers pump just before they go to bed, at about 11pm, and then plan to pump again at about 4am, then restart more frequent pumping later in the morning. Some mothers find it really psychologically difficult to set alarms to pump for a baby who is sick or cannot feed, especially if they are not with their child (if they are on PICU for instance). One tried and tested, gentle way to wake up is to drink a very large glass of water right before bed. The mother will almost certainly wake up to use the bathroom and can pump before going back to sleep.

It's a good idea to recommend pumping until the milk either stops flowing/dripping or becomes very slow. The rate of milk production is driven by the degree of breast emptying, so pumping until the breast is well drained, is wise. Utilising what we know about milk volumes from Chapter 2, one suggestion is to try to pump through more than one let-down, remembering that the average number of let-downs per feed is four. If a mother pumps through four let-downs, they can be fairly confident that they are draining their breasts well, though of course everyone is different, and mothers are the experts on their own breasts and milk supply.

There may be times when a mother does not have time to do a full pump. At these times, it's still better to pump a little – most of the milk removed will happen towards the beginning of the feed/ pumping session, so even pumping for five minutes would remove some milk and keep milk synthesis high, preventing the build-up of the small whey protein FIL (Feedback Inhibitor of Lactation) which will eventually downregulate the milk supply.

Supporting mothers of older children with pumping

Most research related to pumping relates to younger infants, and indeed, when an infant is under six months, the milk volumes are usually larger (Yeung, 2019). With the introduction of solid foods, milk volumes very slowly reduce as food increasingly becomes a more significant part of the child's calorie and nutritional intake. The research into supporting pumping with younger infants is also relevant because the milk supply of a very young child is more vulnerable. Once milk supply is more established, it is common for many mothers to find that their supply is more robust and can tolerate a few longer breaks in between pumping (Wambach and Spencer, 2021).

However, just because pumping to protect the milk supply for an exclusively breast milk fed baby which may be more susceptible to infrequent or ineffective expressing, does not mean that pumping for an older child with a more established milk supply is *easier*. Many mothers have told me about a few distinct problems with pumping for their older child who is unwell:

- There is an assumption that anyone can just pump, and in fact, many mothers hear the suggestion 'why don't you *just* pump' as if it was that easy.
- As milk volumes decrease, it can be much harder to express these small volumes.

- When milk regulation switches to autocrine control (regulated by removal of milk) as opposed to endocrine control (when hormones regulate milk supply to a much greater extent), many mothers find that pumping is harder work.

- With lower volumes, there is less sensation of breast fullness, and these mothers seem particularly vulnerable to stress impacting their milk ejection reflex. They don't always get the sense that they need to pump for comfort, and it is easier to 'forget' to pump in a high stress environment without this physical reminder of fullness.

- Very unwell children often need more fluid than can be provided by the relatively small amounts of breast milk that their mothers are able to express. Older children who eat solid food as well do not need the larger volumes that a younger infant consumes, but when critically ill they usually cannot eat solid food, leading to a reliance on liquid calories in the form of large volumes of milk, which may not be possible to produce. This can lead to a loss of confidence and a feeling that these small volumes are unimportant.

I am not aware of *any* research exploring how to support mothers of older infants, toddlers and children who are unwell. These are anecdotal findings based on my work with many parents of older children over the years. As with so many areas within clinical paediatric-focused lactation support, there is an urgent need for more research. But in the meantime, it is wise to remember that not everyone finds pumping easy, and this seems to be particularly prevalent among mothers of older children. It is also a good idea therefore to have realistic expectations of volumes within this group of mothers and children, and reassure mothers of the normalcy of the lower volumes, or how common it is for mothers of older children to struggle to pump, even if they had no problems with pumping in the early weeks, or have been breastfeeding for many years without concerns about low supply. These mothers also need more support and encouragement, as well as more techniques to optimise relaxation and feeling safe. Certainly, many of the suggestions in this chapter will be relevant for these mothers, but they may additionally need some anticipatory guidance about volumes.

Supporting pumping mothers

Perhaps it is an unhelpful truth that on the paediatric ward, we can just go to the storeroom or milk kitchen and select a milk for a child whenever we need it. I sometimes wonder if this makes milk feel 'disposable', easily replaced, or presents a stark contrast between the convenience of going to the cupboard, versus the time and work of pumping. Many mothers have told me that they felt that when they were pumping, it became all about the milk, and not about the process, or about their needs. If staff become fixated on volumes or frequency of feeding, they can lose sight of the effort expended to produce the milk in the first place.

When we think for a moment about the milk, it is not just a white fluid with dynamic living ingredients and calories. There are many aspects of providing breast milk that are unrelated to nutrition and specifically about the act of expressing:

- Time
- Energy
- Discomfort
- Inconvenience
- Sacrifice

Sometimes pumping is a permanent solution. Other times it is an unwilling intervention. Occasionally it is part of a highly complex feeding plan that feels ever-changing. Never assume that pumping is easy, or simple. Pumping mothers, whether short or long-term, need and deserve compassion, understanding and support, and the milk they hand to staff to put in the fridge should be treated with respect. I have sadly heard many mothers say that staff acted like the milk was 'icky', pulling faces when handling it, or treating it in the same way they would treat a bedpan. Some mothers also felt dehumanised when staff focused on the volumes of milk obtained, or worse still, complained about how little space there was in the fridge or freezer thanks to their pumping output. Please always remember that pumping decisions are not always straightforward.

Types of pump

Mothers often ask what type of pump they should use. If they are pumping in the hospital, they may be limited by what is available on the unit. Some mothers are unable to bring their own electric items into hospital because they have not been electric tested. Therefore, some mothers like to keep a manual breast pump just in case the unit or ward breast pumps are all in use. In an ideal world, there would be a designated expressing room within the Paediatric Department for those who desire privacy, with an adequate number of pumps, additional portable pumps for expressing at the bed or cot side and milk storage facilities. If that is impossible then having some manual pumps may be a good emergency option.

In general, the best substitute for an efficiently feeding baby is a powerful, double electric pump, and there are many WHO code compliant pump manufacturers who already supply pumps to neonatal units. I have provided links to some pump manufacturers in the appendix. Some mothers like to use the pump to express one side at a time, while others prefer double-pumping.

Whichever pump is used, it's important that the pump funnel, or flange is the right fit for the mother. Not everyone's nipples are the same size. If you use a flange that is too wide in diameter, it can suck some of the surrounding areolar tissue into the funnel and this can cause bruising, burns and pain. If the funnel is too narrow in diameter, it can chafe on the shank of the nipple which creates a friction wound. Either too small or too large, a flange will probably reduce milk supply and milk output due to pain. It's best to stock a variety of flange sizes – all major pump manufacturers produce flanges in a variety of sizes, and it's a good idea to check with the mother about whether the pump is comfortable. Sometimes mothers put up with discomfort thinking that this is just the way it is, without realising that there might be a solution. One mother I spoke to was given a flange that was the wrong fit and ended up with an open wound on her nipple that became infected. Having the wrong equipment is not a trivial problem – it is really important that equipment is fit for purpose.

Stage fright

I'll be coming back to some specific techniques for getting the most out of the pump. But first of all, it's important to consider 'stage fright'. For some mothers, the pressure to pump certain volumes, or to build up a stash of milk, or get one feed ahead of themselves, is high. Remember that for many parents, a major priority for their babies is to grow and gain weight. This, of course, is directly linked to milk intake, and many mothers feel this acutely. As well as this, many parents are very concerned about their baby's health and wellbeing. Mothers pumping milk for babies or children who are critically unwell is very stressful. The psychological pressure that many mothers face is huge, and this can have a negative effect on their milk ejection reflex, and thus, their milk volumes.

A really common phenomenon is for a mother to try to express, and then find that very little milk comes. Often, I have worked with mothers who watch the pump closely, waiting anxiously for drops. When a mother feeds her baby, the process is a lot more automatic, because they have a relationship with their baby. Because they love their baby, and oxytocin is, among many other things, the hormone of love, the milk ejection reflex is instinctive and predictable.

Pumping and nursing a baby are two entirely different things. Oxytocin is the hormone that initiates the milk ejection reflex, and that hormone is inhibited by stress. It's very common for the pressure to produce a certain amount of milk to interfere with being able to produce that milk. It doesn't mean the milk has 'dried up'. It's just that this can be quite a 'shy' process.

Some simple strategies to combat stage fright include suggesting relaxation techniques such as progressive muscle relaxation, listening to music or meditation. Some mothers like mindfulness activities, repeating affirmations or visualising milk flowing and pouring. I often see a blanket recommendation to have a photo of the baby or an item of the baby or child's clothing nearby, as scent can be a powerful trigger. Just be open minded though – I've known many mothers to find this stress-inducing, as it seems to remind them of how much pressure they are under to make milk. It can also be far from relaxing to look at a photo of their critically sick child, and I have known many mothers describe this as triggering. If this strategy works, that's great, but be aware it's not a technique that will be suitable for absolutely everyone.

For mothers who do not find this helpful, I've found several alternative techniques work really well. Firstly, you could try some distraction. I've had success with just chatting to mothers about entirely unrelated things that are meaningful to them – whether that is the tattoo on their arm, their favourite TV show, or their cat. I sometimes recommend comedy. Getting parents to laugh is a great way to help them relax. If you're not a stand-up comedian, just suggest watching a comedy show on YouTube.

You could also try some reverse psychology. Setting the bar really low by saying something like *'now, this isn't the same thing as direct breastfeeding, and it can take some practice, so don't worry about how much milk you get, it's just about practising the technique'* can really help. The chances are, if you set the bar low, the mother will exceed their own expectations and then this will become a positive self-fulfilling prophecy. Also, try to recommend not watching the drips or the milk level in the bottle constantly. It's fine to watch from time to time when you're altering position to see if that yields more milk, but generally, it's not relaxing to watch milk dripping, similar to the old adage *'a watched pot never boils'*. Some mothers find putting a sock over the pump bottle so they cannot see the milk is a helpful technique - just be careful it doesn't overflow while you're not watching!

Finally, you could throw in some massage – while not everyone enjoys touch, many people find touch empathic, soothing and it can stimulate oxytocin. If there is a partner around that is ideal, but if not, you could demonstrate how to roll your shoulders, press the acupressure point (GB21) which is found about halfway along the clavicle, or squeeze the base of the joint between the thumb and forefinger (LI4) where there is another oxytocin pressure point which has been found to be effective by many proponents of traditional medicine and one study found to be effective in increasing milk volumes (Hajian et al, 2021).

Many mothers find it helps to have a little routine before pumping, such as having a drink or a snack or listening to an audiobook. Importantly, eating and drinking will not make more milk, but on the other hand, being hungry or thirsty may increase physiological stress, which may make pumping harder due to an inhibited oxytocin response.

Maximising pumping efficiency

Whichever way a mother is pumping, it's important to know how to get the most milk for the least amount of time and effort. A mother is much more likely to commit to pumping if it can be made as supportive and easy as possible. At low milk volumes – for example, either when a parent is re-lactating after stopping breastfeeding, or before the onset of lactogenesis II, hand expressing is much more effective than using a pump (Morton, 2009, Morton et al, 2012, Parker et al, 2012). However, even after the onset of copious milk production, it's still important for the mother to know how to use their hands when they pump.

A lot of people don't know how to get the most out of their pumping session. The way we pump has been shown in some studies by Dr. Jane Morton and colleagues to directly impact milk output (Morton et al, 2014).

There is a link to a video by Dr. Morton in the appendix, but in brief, hands-on pumping involves pushing the pump flange gently into the chest wall, and then rotating the pump around to empty more of the milk ducts. While doing this, the mother can also use some breast compressions – which is where you place your hand in a C shape and squeeze and hold the breast. They can also gently massage and instinctively feel for areas of fullness. Finally, they could try the so-called *'milk shake'* coined by Dr. Christina Smillie, which is where the parent removes the pump, and literally wobbles their breast tissue, then re-applies the pump. It might sound ridiculous, but milk fat is very sticky, and some physical (gentle) shaking can help to move it down the milk duct. Just make sure that the mother knows that whatever they do, it should never be painful – we're not trying to scare the milk out! If the mother does use massage, this should be light pressure only (the kind of pressure you would use to stroke a kitten). Firm kneading or massage with electric toothbrushes and so on has not been found to be helpful, and Dr Katrina Mitchell, who is a breast surgeon and IBCLC, advises avoiding firm massage of the breast. Her blog provides really helpful additional information on the explanatory breast physiology to support this recommendation: https://physicianguidetobreastfeeding.org/mythbusters/massage/

Preparation and cleaning

When it comes to hygiene, there is not a huge amount of preparatory work to be done, though please refer to your local guidelines and remember that extra precautions may be necessary for extremely vulnerable or immunocompromised children. There is no need to wash the nipples or breast, but hands should always be washed. The pump will probably come with a compatible plastic container/bottle that can be used to store the milk once pumped. In a hospital setting, these are usually sterile single use containers, and therefore there is usually no need to clean them. If the mother is pumping at home, they may collect their milk in a sturdy milk storage bag, or a hard plastic or glass container.

Preparation, storage and sterilisation guidelines will vary with local policy, so check with your policies and infection control documents to see what is recommended in your unit. I'm mindful that some professionals may be caring for severely compromised infants, while others are not – so a blanket statement on cleaning and storage is not appropriate.

The mother can start with some gentle breast stroking and nipple rolling. I often find that mothers feel strange about this, perhaps because they think it is for relaxation – like a back rub or a foot massage. If mothers believe that pre-pumping touch is for relaxation purposes, and it *isn't* relaxing, they may opt out of doing it. I always explain that while it's fine if it *does* feel relaxing, this is not really the purpose. In fact, it can feel odd to some mothers to touch their own breasts (though it is a great opportunity to educate about breast self-exams!). The main reason to recommend this practice is to stimulate prolactin, which is triggered through touch, and partially replicates what the infant would do if they were able to directly feed.

If the milk supply is well established, start by electric pumping using the hands-on pumping technique, and then finish with hand expression. In the first few days after birth, or if re-lactating, start with hand expressing.

Outside the hospital environment, or if the mother is re-using the pump parts, these should be completely taken apart after use and washed in hot soapy water. For at-risk or immunocompromised infants, the parts should then be sterilised. Even though human milk is actively phagocytic, with live white cells ingesting any bacteria, if a child is neutropenic, it is a good idea to reduce any potential risks.

Storing milk

There are a bewildering variety of nuances when it comes to milk storage, and again, please refer to your local policy or guidelines. Storage recommendations basically depend on the temperature you intend to store the milk at. Unless a mother is pumping in a very warm environment, freshly expressed milk can be stored at room temperature for four to eight hours, depending on which guideline or study you read, and again, you may wish to be more conservative if the child is very unwell. It can also be stored in the fridge. Some texts recommend that expressed breast milk can be stored for up to 96 hours, and other studies recommend that for compromised infants and children that we suggest a more conservative two days (Steele, 2018). Raw human milk does not keep for as long as pasteurised milk, and just like any other mammal's milk, it will smell rancid if it's past its best. Extra precautions may also be deemed necessary when a child is immunocompromised.

Milk can also be frozen, but the exact amount of time it can be kept depends on the temperature of the freezer, and how often the freezer door tends to be opened. In a freezer above a fridge, three months is usually cited at the conservative end of the estimate, and in a deep freeze or chest freezer that isn't opened as frequently, six months, and even up to 12 months is tolerable (Eglash et al, 2017).

When milk is frozen, it's a good idea to recommend not filling the container up to the brim, as milk has a high water content and will expand when frozen.

From a practical point of view, it is also a good idea to store milk in a variety of volumes, and if in doubt about how much milk a baby will drink in one feed, store in very small quantities to prevent wasting milk. Many mothers have told me despairingly that a 200ml bottle of expressed milk was defrosted in order to provide 20ml of milk. It is devastating to a mother who has painstakingly expressed to see the majority of their milk discarded. It is therefore worth some anticipatory guidance to mothers and parents about storing milk in a variety of sized containers.

While we're on the subject of volumes, it's a good idea to manage expectations about milk volume with mothers who are new to pumping. You may remember from Chapter 2 that all breasts have different storage capacities. The average amount of milk produced for a baby aged one to six months is 750ml. Some women will need to pump 35ml from each breast, ten times per day to produce this. Others will be able to pump less frequently as their storage capacity is much greater. If we hand the mother who can only pump 20ml from her left breast and 50ml from her right breast a 250ml bottle, she may feel completely inadequate. But on the other hand, if a mother is regularly producing 200ml from each breast, handing her a 50ml bottle is frustrating. The solution is to ensure that mothers know that all breasts make milk at different rates, and to offer a selection of sized containers, asking them to choose what is most appropriate for them.

In hospital, most people use the baby's hospital stickers as these already have the baby's name, date of birth and hospital number so that milk stored in a communal fridge does not get mixed up. Someone will just need to add the date and time of expression. You could also give them a roll of stickers so that they can label their own milk and save them from frequently asking for stickers, which can be frustrating - especially when staff are busy or it's the middle of the night. One mother I spoke to was understandably furious when all her milk was thrown out because it did not have her child's ID sticker on it, despite the fact that she was the only breastfeeding mother on the ward and the milk could only have been hers. Please make this part of your job, so that parents are not put in these impossible situations!

When giving milk to a baby, it's best to use freshly expressed milk first. If infants are only getting occasional feeds of stored milk, it is perhaps less significant that some nutrients are reduced due to storage. But if an infant is not able to directly breastfeed at all, we should make the best possible effort to preserve nutrients. Milk that has been frozen is lower in immunologic properties and Vitamin C, though it does retain its antibacterial properties in the fridge for several days (Weaver et al, 2019).

If fresh milk is not available, frozen milk still provides optimal nutrition for the child. It can be thawed overnight in the fridge, at room temperature, or in a hurry it can be defrosted under warm running water or placed in a bowl of warm water. Some babies prefer milk slightly warm, while others are happy to drink it at room temperature. When milk is stored, it will separate, with the cream fraction rising to the top. This is normal for any unhomogenized milk, and the milk can be gently swirled to redistribute the cream.

Once milk is thawed, it can be kept in the fridge for 24 hours, but if a baby has started to feed from a bottle, it should be used within one to two hours, and leftover milk should not be re-frozen – which is why storing it in small quantities may be a pragmatic way of reducing waste.

When mothers choose to exclusively pump

There are many reasons why a mother may end up choosing or needing to exclusively express their milk. They may do this from the beginning, following a struggle with their infant – perhaps due to anatomical challenges or dysfunctional suck, because they themselves are sick, are experiencing nursing aversion, or because they do not enjoy breastfeeding but still want their child to benefit from their milk.

I've run into mothers whose older child is sick, and they choose to express milk for their older child, as well as continue to nurse their younger child. It's important to be aware that everyone has a different story and a reason why they exclusively pump. I'm not suggesting that this is the most common reason but do be aware that for some parents it could be deeply personal and due to body or gender dysphoria, previous sexual abuse, violence or trauma.

The bottom line – compassion is needed at all times, and we should value all milk, regardless of how it is given, how exclusively, or in what volume (Felice et al, 2017).

If you are supporting a mother who is exclusively expressing, try to manage how the baby receives the milk by giving milk that is as fresh as possible. This not only preserves the nutrients, but also means babies are given milk that is appropriate from a circadian point of view as well. Human milk mirrors maternal blood hormone levels and the glandular mammary tissue makes specific immunoglobulins in response to infant-mother immune cross talk. This is slightly harder when an infant is not suckling, as the breast does not receive infant signals. So, encourage plenty of skin-to-skin, cuddles and nurturing to get as much immunological crosstalk as you can.

The other thing to remember with exclusive expressing is that different techniques and strategies will work for different mothers. You will find that some mothers need to pump more frequently, whereas others can get away with less frequent expressing. Some mothers may get better results from double pumping, whereas others do better when they pump one side at a time, using their hands and maximising efficiency. Some will need additional strategies to maintain or increase their milk supply, or a different type of pump to better meet their needs. Some mothers do better with hand expressing instead of using a pump, and vice versa. Basically - keep an open mind – everyone is different.

Increasing milk supply

Some mothers struggle to maintain their milk supply either if they are not exclusively breastfeeding, such as when they are feeding a baby with an inborn error of metabolism which may affect their ability to be exclusively breastfed, their baby feeds inefficiently for whatever reason, or they are exclusively pumping by choice. Some mothers find that their milk supply seems to dip when their older child is unexpectedly seriously unwell. Often the volumes produced for an older baby or toddler are naturally lower, and not all mothers pump as a regular part of their feeding journey. Therefore, for some, acute serious or critical illness is a risky time for their milk supply as they may not be able to pump easily. Other mothers want to increase milk production or re-lactate when they learn that their infant is unwell. My systematic review found that an ill baby was a big motivator to continue providing human milk (re-lactation resources in the Appendix).

If a mother wishes to re-lactate – this is to initiate a milk supply after having stopped - the success of this depends on how long after they have stopped that they re-start, how exclusively they were feeding when they stopped, and whether there were any underlying problems in the first place. Generally, the shorter the interval between stopping and restarting, and the more exclusively they were feeding before they stopped, the better their chances.

For anyone trying to increase their supply, either from drops, a partial supply or a nearly full supply, it is important to rule out any underlying causes of low supply. For the most part, low milk supply is due to insufficient stimulation or milk removal in the early days, often a combination of infant and parental factors. However, sometimes low milk supply is caused by or related to breast or chest/thoracic surgery, Sheehan's Syndrome, infertility, endocrine dysfunction, such as thyroid disorder, or breast hypoplasia – a rare but nevertheless significant cause of primary hypolactation. If these issues are raised during a more thorough breastfeeding assessment, then it is worth making sure the mother gets support from skilled professionals who can help to unpick this. This may include an IBCLC, as well as their medical provider if hormone dysfunction is suspected.

For mothers of sick children, common causes of very low supply are feeding pauses, as well as acute stress and trauma. Therefore, assuming underlying causes have been ruled out, it's a good idea to reduce stress and difficulty for the family. This is often easier said than done for a parent of a sick child. The mothers themselves may be best placed to think of practical solutions that could potentially make their life easier. Systematically working out what the sources of stress are, and then trying to creatively problem solve to reduce the *number* or severity of stresses may lessen their mental load and stress levels. For example, there may be worries about employment that would be helped by an official letter of support from the hospital. There may be anxieties about other children, or practical problems such as eating, pet care and tasks at home. Sometimes during acute stress, parents find it hard to think in this systematic way, so a nudge to think logically can be helpful.

If a child has been critically unwell and unable to directly breastfeed, it is likely that with patience, perseverance and calm, the child can be returned to breastfeeding once they are clinically stable. I have met many families who have found that this only happened once they were discharged home. The implication of this is that families may need some pragmatic, realistic anticipatory guidance to help manage their expectations. Milk supply can recover, but it does sometimes take some time.

Often the mainstay of increasing milk supply will be pumping and hand expressing, so you can utilise all the tools we discussed for maximising pumping efficiency. Often mothers are put off pumping frequently because they assume they will need to pump for 30-40 minutes every 3 hours.

It can be a lot more realistic for some mothers to think about power pumping or cluster pumping or making the pumping plan more flexible instead. I've met many mothers who pump three times a day for 30 minutes, because they assume that less time than this is not beneficial if they cannot fully drain the breast. But remember, the rate of milk synthesis is driven by breast fullness. So, just doing 5 to 10 minutes of pumping will remove a little bit of milk, and thus maintain a faster rate of milk production. I often explain that initially, when you are trying to build your supply back up again, it is arguably better to pump 10 to 12 times a day for 10 to 15 minutes, instead of three to four times a day for 40 minutes. This often takes the pressure off, and mothers feel more optimistic about being able to squeeze in more frequent expressing sessions. Once milk supply begins to increase, of course, draining the breast well is also important, but it would still be better to pump for a short amount of time, rather than to skip a pumping session entirely.

Some mothers like the idea of power pumping. There are various ways to do this, but they are all based on the idea of pumping very frequently with short breaks in between. So, a mother may pump for 10 minutes, then rest for 10 minutes, then repeat. Other mothers 'switch pump'. They pump one side for 10 minutes, then the other side and repeat until the milk stops flowing, following that up with hand expressing. There are some resources in the appendix on power pumping.

I sometimes recommend leaving the pump out for four hours at room temperature, and just pumping for five minutes every time they pass the pump. At the end of the four hours, put the collected milk in a bottle and refrigerate. This works well for mothers with very low supply, whose milk would barely line the bottom of the bottle. It is less demoralising to collect it up over several pumping sessions. Feel free to experiment, suggest a variety of strategies, and see what works for an individual mother. Often, a rigid set of instructions can feel off putting, so make sure that parents know how they can tailor the suggestions to find what works for them.

Mothers are often told to drink more if they are trying to increase their supply. There is no evidence for this, unless they are clinically dehydrated. In fact, drinking too much water can make parents feel unwell. Drinking to thirst is still the best advice in this regard.

Other mothers are interested in galactagogues – or substances to increase milk supply. There are three main types – pharmacological galactagogues, herbal galactagogues, and foods.

Domperidone

The main pharmacological treatment is domperidone, a dopamine antagonist, which means that it will result in increased prolactin secretion from the pituitary gland. Most studies find that it increases milk supply, although not all studies show that it increases milk supply drastically. Prolactin levels are not necessarily related to overall milk production, however. Levels of prolactin are highest in pregnancy, and then fall. They drop quite significantly at around 6 to 12 weeks, with no corresponding drop in milk supply, so it is clear that it isn't all about prolactin. However, if blood prolactin levels fall to within the non-pregnant range, it may be that they are low enough to reduce milk supply. It would not be unreasonable to check the blood prolactin levels to see if this is a problem.

A large trial found that it appears to be safe for short term use (Smolina et al, 2016). However, it is an off-label use of the drug, and there were some concerns raised some years ago about very rare but serious cardiac side effects in patients with a pre-existing cardiac condition, or who were taking drugs that prolonged the Q-T interval. For this reason, it became unpopular for a while. It is not licensed in the US, though is still prescribed as an aid to lactation in the UK and other parts of the world, particularly among mothers of preterm babies, though as it is an off-label use of the drug, medical practitioners have to be willing to accept medico-legal responsibility for prescribing it.

It's important to note that domperidone does not work like a magic bullet. There is no substitute for effective, frequent milk removal. So even if the mother is taking domperidone, they will need to be pumping regularly and effectively.

Herbs

Herbal galactagogues have become increasingly popular, and many people equate herbal or natural with 'safe'. However, just because something doesn't require a prescription, doesn't necessarily make it safe. There is very little evidence for many of the herbs that are commonly used, and some trials have shown conflicting results. One of the most well-known herbal galactagogues is fenugreek, which is not recommended by many IBCLCs due to its very patchy evidence base and many side effects. Herbs can interact with existing conditions or medications, and it is always best to check with a doctor or pharmacist. Some herbs may also cause allergic reactions.

Other herbs may be chemically similar to prescription medication, such as goats' rue, which has a similar effect to metformin. Others may cause hypoglycaemia or act as diuretics. An excellent resource is *Making More Milk*, by Diana West and Lisa Marasco (2019) which has lots of practical tools for increasing milk supply, and a comprehensive table of herbal galactagogues with indications, contraindications and any known evidence base supporting their use.

Caution with herbal recommendations is especially important for infants who are unwell, have altered or immature metabolic or excretory pathways. It's also important to remember for infants in the first to third days of life as there are large spaces between the lactocyte cell junctions prior to the onset of lactogenesis II when the lactocytes swelling with milk causes the closure of these tight junctions. This means that during this time, drugs may more readily enter the milk, and in higher concentrations than may be found at a later stage of lactation.

It's worth mentioning that drugs pass into human milk at highly variable rates depending on many aspects of pharmacokinetics. Many mothers are indiscriminately told they cannot breastfeed because of a medication they are taking, or told to 'pump and dump'. Most of the time, this is unnecessary, though there are a few drugs that are incompatible with breastfeeding - please check some of the reputable lactation pharmacy sources (do not rely on the British National

Formulary!). It's also worth knowing that babies are more exposed to drugs via the placenta than they are via milk, so if a needed drug was felt to be safe in pregnancy, there isn't a logical argument for withholding it after birth. However, it is worth checking with an experienced pharmacist, or consulting one of the excellent drugs in human milk textbooks as the data for hundreds of different drugs is known. Thomas Hale's book is excellent (Hale and Rowe, 2016), and Wendy Jones (2018) is also a fountain of information. You can also access *Hale online*, *The Breastfeeding Network* drugs in breast milk factsheets and website, *Lactmed* and the *Lactation Pharmacist* on Facebook to look drugs up and ask questions.

In general, there are some characteristics of drugs that are associated with a greater level of confidence in respect of their safety. These include drugs where the relative infant dose is less than 10% of the maternal dose, as well as drugs that are poorly orally bioavailable – such as vancomycin. Drugs with a short half-life will be excreted rapidly, so pumping or feeding can potentially be timed around the administration of these drugs – for example general anaesthetics are excreted fairly rapidly, so as soon as they no longer feel groggy, there will be very little drug left in their system. If a drug is highly protein-bound, it means there isn't much free drug – this is the case for most penicillins. Drugs that are lipid soluble may pass more readily into milk, especially if they are also of low molecular weight, so choosing a drug that has low lipid solubility is better for infants, as are drugs that do not cross the blood-brain barrier.

Finally – it's an obvious point, but just because something is safe, doesn't mean it won't have other effects on milk and milk supply – take care with medications such as oestrogen and the combined oral contraceptive pill, as well as many cold and flu remedies that contain pseudoephedrine. It's worth checking that a mother isn't taking any of these medications before working on milk supply, as cessation of this medication may spontaneously improve milk production.

Foods

Foods may seem like the safest option. But just as with herbs, there is very little robust evidence, and some foods may actually reduce supply – such as peppermint, sage and parsley, though this is limited to anecdotal evidence (Johnson et al, 2020). There are also many myths about foods that are perceived to be lactogenic, without concrete evidence.

I'm mindful though, that just because there is limited research, there may be traditional customs that have simply not been explored by researchers yet. In saying that there is little evidence, I am not saying that I disregard or disrespect people's cultural beliefs about foods that may support milk production. We will, as with so many other areas within lactation, have to wait for more research.

Be careful – as some foods have medicinal properties, and again, I highly recommend West and Marasco (2019) for a more in-depth discussion of not only foods but also herbs that may or may not have an impact on milk supply. Oats are probably the most well-known galactagogue and have been used by the dairy industry for many decades to increase the milk production of cows. Other foods, such as dill, fennel and alfalfa also have a small amount of evidence that they may modestly increase milk supply or the MER, but take care with allergies, as alfalfa sprouts are from the legume family. Nettle and dandelion are often taken as herbal tea preparations, and hops can be taken in capsule form.

The bottom line is that like herbs and even medications to increase milk supply, there is no substitute for frequent, effective milk removal. In addition, there is an argument that focusing on maternal diet can lead many mothers to believe that their milk will not be good quality or quantity because their diet is not perfect. In fact, this is a myth that has been used by the formula milk industry for decades to undermine maternal confidence. So while some foods may have some anecdotal lactogenic properties, we should keep a sensible level of perspective about this.

Using donor human milk

Donor milk provision is well established among high-risk neonatal patients, and some milk banks provide donor human milk to mothers going through chemotherapy or following mastectomy who cannot breastfeed. However, there is an argument for making donor milk available to full term infants and children – particularly those who may be vulnerable either because of a specific gut condition, or those susceptible to opportunistic respiratory infections, which breastfed children are less likely to experience, as well as conditions which affect the immune system.

Donor human milk has been shown to motivate and encourage mothers to provide their own milk in stressful situations in the neonatal intensive care unit. You can find a list of donor milk resources and milk banks in the Appendix. Providing donor milk is often perceived as supportive of a mother's own efforts to express, rather than feeling like failure when formula is needed to supplement breast milk production (Kantorowska et al, 2016). A recent study has also demonstrated the many positive impacts on parent's wellbeing of being given the opportunity to use donor human milk. Aside from increased immune protection, the experience of being respected, listened to and cared for when it comes to infant feeding decisions protects parental wellbeing (Brown and Shenker, 2022).

While some hospitals may provide donor milk to term babies in certain circumstances, for example hypoglycaemia (Ferrarello et al, 2019), there is less established practice of providing it to term babies or older babies in general. There are currently no definitive guidelines available, though this is moving in a positive direction, with many milk banks providing screened donor milk on a case-by-case basis. The Heart Milk Bank is also working to develop plans to increase the provision of donor human milk into paediatrics. Some clinicians may be concerned about infection risk, but this would be extremely unlikely with pasteurised donor milk since the donors are screened and the milk is treated.

A recent case series explored the feasibility and outcomes of using donor milk to term babies who had been abandoned at birth and exposed to HIV. Anecdotally, these babies seemed to be buffered from complications such as faltering growth, diarrhoeal illness and opportunistic infections (Reimers et al, 2018; McCune and Perrin, 2021; Bramer et al, 2021; Griffin et al, 2022). Clearly more research is needed to explore the feasibility of donor human milk use in sick and medically complex infants, but in theory at least, this should be considered a viable option for some children.

I know of several mothers anecdotally who have shared raw milk informally and have found this to be protective of their mental health at a difficult time when their own milk supply dipped. The children concerned also all universally had good outcomes. I also know of identical twins who wet nursed each other's children, including one child who had cancer. Open-mindedness is key here. While there may not be research currently to prove that this is safe, we sometimes need to ask the question - why not? Ultimately, if a mother has made an informed decision, it is their choice, but I do wish we had more research to reassure those who may be sceptical! Furthermore, to play devil's advocate, if screened donor milk is not available, then informal milk sharing may be the most acceptable choice for a family who holds strong views about giving their child formula. There are risks with sharing unpasteurised raw milk, but there are also risks of giving formula. We need to accept that if we do not provide donor milk, informal milk sharing may be chosen by families, with or without the knowledge of the medical practitioners involved. The sooner we can scale provision of donor milk into paediatrics the better.

Triple feeding

Triple feeding is the term used when mothers are breastfeeding, expressing their milk to give to their baby (often via a supplementer device or a bottle), as well as topping up with infant formula or donor milk – the term obviously comes from the fact that parents are feeding their baby in three ways. It's definitely not something most people would choose to do. It's hard work, and very time consuming (Lucas et al, 2014; Briere et al, 2015; Noble et al, 2018; McCue and Stulberger, 2019; Elder et al, 2022), but there are some common scenarios that make this feeding choice more likely:

- A sleepy baby who is not feeding effectively, common among babies with jaundice.
- Babies with excessive weight loss, who have been put on a feeding plan.
- Low milk supply/poor infant weight gain.
- Late preterm babies, who sometimes need a bit more time to be able to complete an entire feed at the breast.
- Babies with underlying medical complexity.
- Babies with higher calorie needs.

In my experience, triple feeding and feeding plans usually have a back story that goes back to the very first day. The all-too-familiar tale is of a baby who *seemed* to be feeding, only to be weighed a couple of days later and for a weight loss of more than 10% to be discovered. This is why it is so important to be able to recognise effective feeding in the first few feeds and hours. The trick with a triple feeding situation is to have a sustainable plan. It boils down, once again, to this:

1. Keep the baby fed (preferably in a style supportive of breastfeeding, using expressed milk, donor milk, or formula).
2. Protect the milk supply (and possibly increase it if necessary).
3. Figure out the underlying cause and make a bespoke plan to help the mother achieve their goals, bearing the cause in mind.
4. Transition the baby back to direct breastfeeding (if desired).

If there is not a plan, then triple feeding can go on for longer than necessary. If formula is involved, then unless there is an active management plan to increase the maternal milk supply, then the supply will almost certainly take a hit. Sometimes using formula is a necessary part of this process, but it does rather complicate breastfeeding in a number of ways. We also know that maternal feeding goals are important, and not meeting them can lead to grief, regret and sadness (Brown, 2018; 2019). For these reasons, sometimes it helps to have a strategic plan to return to breastfeeding and reduce the top ups.

Step 1: Keep the baby fed.

This may sound simple enough. But the devil is in the details. It's not enough to simply give mothers an exact number of millilitres to get their baby to drink every few hours. Parents need to know *how* to feed this milk to their baby as well. There are a couple of things that can go wrong here.

Firstly, if the baby is being supplemented with a bottle, it is essential that the parents know how to pace the feed, and feed responsively. This slows the feed down, helps the baby to manage the flow rate, and prevents the baby from becoming frustrated with the slower flow from the breast. At the breast, a baby is more in control of the flow of milk, and the flow rate changes throughout the feed, according to fullness, infant suckling, and individual anatomical factors.

Remember you don't have to recommend a bottle. There are other options – such as supplementer, bridge device (this is a kit that combines a nipple shield attached to a tube, with a syringe, in order that a baby may be supplemented with small amounts at the breast – it is particularly useful for infants who have become used to a bottle), cup, spoon, or finger feed. It's worth involving an experienced lactation professional, breastfeeding counsellor or IBCLC if your client/patient wants to use any of these options. Clearly, not all options are suitable for every child with a medical complexity, so collaborative, respectful and open-minded brainstorming between clinical and lactation advocates may be required.

The second problem I run into is the baby who is fussy at the breast. One scenario I've seen play out over and over again is the baby who is not effectively latching or becomes distressed at the breast. Often, understandably, mothers give up, as they hate to see their child getting upset and the baby has a bottle. The problem is that if we count this unsuccessful attempt as a legitimate feed, and do not protect the milk supply by pumping, then the supply will quickly dwindle.

A better way is often to make sure the baby is calm and not super hungry. This way, they're more likely to have an effective feed. In practice, offering a small amount of their top-up can calm a hungry baby so that they can then feed effectively. Christina Smillie MD IBCLC coined the term *'finish at the breast'* – although of course, many mothers find themselves instinctively trying this when they realise that breast first doesn't work so well.

Step 2: Protect the milk supply.

This is the part of triple feeding that most often gets missed. There is a narrow window of opportunity to calibrate the milk supply in the early days and weeks. If we miss that window, then it can be much harder (though not impossible) to increase milk production. Often the focus is on ensuring the baby is fed, which of course is the priority, but we cannot take our eyes off the vulnerable milk supply. If milk supply is established in a child who is older than 4-6 weeks, then even if it reduces due to acute illness or medical complexity, it is usually possible to return to exclusive breastfeeding. However, it is still far easier to protect the milk supply to avoid the mother having to work hard to get the milk volumes back to their previous status.

To protect the milk supply you will need to ensure the mother knows to remove milk - either with the baby, the pump, hand expressing, or possibly all three.

An effectively feeding child is the obvious first choice. If the child is keen and willing to breastfeed, then recommend responsive feeding. If the baby is *not* feeding effectively, then the mother may benefit from some support to optimise feeding, including:

- Watch the baby for deep, active suckling with rhythmic jaw movements.
- Listen for audible swallows.
- Watch the baby's tone and posture, including their hands. A baby who looks relaxed and is obviously drinking is reassuring. A baby who is wriggly, squirmy, fussy, and pulling off and crying is less so.
- Try some breast compressions to increase the flow and fat content of milk.
- If the baby is not feeding, or not feeding often or effectively enough, then pumping is essential – at least 8-12 times in 24 hours.

Step 3: Figure out the underlying cause.

It sounds pretty obvious, but different people have different and unique problems. If we adopt a cookie cutter strategy with triple feeding, it's unlikely to be successful for everyone. Understanding the root cause is much more likely to work well. When working with a family, spend some time listening to their story, hearing about the first few days, as well as asking some specific questions. This will help you to work out whether the low weight gain is due to:

1. Primary maternal factors.
2. Combination of infant and maternal factors.
3. Infant issues only.

I usually start by trying to rule out primary lactation problems. As briefly covered in Chapter 3, these include breast or chest/thoracic surgery (including cosmetic), trauma, scars and anatomical problems. It also includes assessing for signs of breast hypoplasia. I also ask about endocrine problems such as fertility and thyroid problems or diabetes. Finally, it's important to know about breast pathology, either historic or current. You may need to involve a more experienced lactation advocate here if this feels a long way from your knowledge base.

The next part of the detective work is to rule out infant issues. The best way to do this is by watching the baby feed. I cannot tell you how many times I have been to a family who have been told by numerous health professionals that the latch looks 'fine'. The difference between a suboptimal and an optimal latch can look subtle to a less experienced eye.

Almost all the time, there are improvements that can be made to optimise the effectiveness of the feeding. Review the baby's tongue, palate, tone and overall wellbeing and either refer or practice watchful waiting, as the situation dictates.

A combination of maternal and infant factors is the most likely scenario. Usually, this situation arises because although there is the potential for a full milk supply, something has happened in the early days to jeopardise breastfeeding. The less effectively the baby feeds, the less milk they remove. Often the baby loses weight, and simultaneously the milk supply can either dwindle, or the mother can become uncomfortable with engorgement or sore nipples from a shallow latch.

When we know what the underlying problem is, we can target the treatment. It might be to improve the latch. It might be to increase supply. It might be to get the baby healthy again. Whatever it is, the goal is to figure it out and make a plan that addresses the underlying problem(s).

Step 4: Transition the baby back to the breast.

Because triple feeding is not sustainable for the majority of people, most mothers need or want to move away from it as soon as possible. There may be many ways to do this, but this is often what I suggest:

- Firstly, the baby should be gaining weight consistently. 20-30g per day (or individually appropriate amounts based on their age/condition) and two to three yellow stools in the first 6 weeks (fewer stools may be normal for older babies and children). The basics are important.

- Then, if the milk supply is increasing and the baby is gaining weight, we can move on...

- Consider reducing the formula component by 30-40ml in total over 24 hours (not per feed!). We don't want to put the baby at risk. Reducing the formula a little bit will challenge the milk supply by the infant feeding more frequently, but not risk their health. If these volumes feel wildly inappropriate for the clinical situation you are encountering, then of course make adjustments using your clinical judgement.

- In practice, this could be one entire top up feed that is abandoned, or you might want to reduce the amount of 3-4 feeds by 10ml.

- You could also consider suggesting the reduction of pumping sessions, so more milk is in the breast, rather than the bottle. In practice this could be abandoning one pumping session, or you could consider doing away with all but two or three tactical pumping sessions.

- While all this is going on, you'll need to keep a careful eye on the baby's behaviour, nappy output and weight gain. The baby's health and well-being are the top priority.

- I normally suggest reducing the formula every three to four days. Most mothers find this less stressful, as it will take the breasts a few days to catch up with the increased demand.

Many people find it is helpful to set time limits. Triple feeding is very tiring, and emotionally draining. If there is an end or a review point in sight, then psychologically it's easier to keep going. I have often worked with my clients for a few days intensively, then we review and find out if the plan is working or not. It is either:

- Beginning to work – we may collectively agree to persevere and review.

- Working so well that we can start reducing the top ups faster.

- Not making much difference – in which case we decide whether to persevere a bit longer or make a sustainable plan to move forward with.

If the mother ends up with that last option, then most people are hugely comforted by the knowledge that they tried everything. They might decide to keep hold of the most meaningful breastfeeds, and bottle feed in between. They might decide that breastfeeding with a supplementer is the way forward. They might decide that they will keep going with expressing and stop breastfeeding. Or they may feel that they will just keep up what they are doing until it comes to a natural end.

There are many possible outcomes that a family may choose. The important thing is to ensure that they have options and can make an informed decision. It is also important to note that there may be disappointment and grief that the mother has to deal with. I would also add that there are many ways to have a successful feeding journey. Often, with compassionate and sensitive communication, even if the outcome was not what the family desired, they can feel a sense of peace if it was handled well.

Test yourself:

1. Which of the following statements is NOT true about maintaining milk production with pumping?

    a. Pumping is easier for a mother.

    b. At certain times, babies may not be able to directly breast feed.

    c. Pumping/expressing is essential to maintain milk supply if a baby is unable to feed.

    d. Parents may need additional support and encouragement.

2. Which of the following strategies may support a parent who is struggling with an inhibited milk ejection reflex?

    a. Privacy.

    b. Relaxation techniques.

    c. Making donor milk an option to reduce the pressure.

    d. All the above.

3. Which of the statements below is most supportive when working with a mother who is attempting to increase milk supply?

    a. Suggest that a mother asks their doctor for a prescription for domperidone.

    b. Encouraging the mother to drink 3 litres of water a day.

    c. Give them a rigid pumping schedule.

    d. Work with the mother to find a combination of pumping strategies that are sustainable.

4. Which of the following is true of galactagogues and medications?

    a. Fenugreek is the safest galactagogue as it has been recommended for many years.

    b. All medications a mother takes will be found in trace amounts in human milk.

    c. Domperidone can be prescribed to all parents whose prolactin levels are found to be low.

    d. Different parents may need a different approach to increasing milk supply, and no drug or herb is necessarily safe for everyone.

Chapter 8

When supplements and feeding pauses are medically necessary.

In practice, it's common that breastfeeding gets disrupted by unnecessary supplementation. However, that doesn't mean that supplementation is *never* necessary. It's important to understand **when** we may need to supplement, **what** to supplement with and **how** to supplement.

The first choice of supplement is the mother's own expressed milk. If an infant has been ineffectively feeding, they may fail to gain weight, but this is not necessarily a reflection of the mother's ability to make milk. It's always worth first considering whether expressing may be an option. If there isn't any expressed milk, then the next choice is donor human milk if this is possible and available. The third choice is a first stage infant formula. With any of the supplemental feedings, there are many options for how to feed the baby, which I will come to shortly.

Most importantly, continue to provide encouragement. It can feel very demoralising when a mother is told they need to supplement. This is often internalised as 'your milk isn't enough' or even '*you* aren't enough' which is obviously hugely discouraging, as well as clearly untrue. Mothers need support to continue in order to meet their feeding goals, and from a practical point of view, they also need to protect their milk supply while the supplement is given.

Medical indication for supplementation

Moving on to think about reasons for supplementation, the most well-known scenario is the baby with clinically significant dehydration or weight loss (beyond the weight loss that we sometimes see at birth). Dehydration can be assessed fairly objectively and managed according to severity. Dehydration is usually classified as:

- Mild (<5% weight loss)
- Moderate (5-10% weight loss)
- Severe (>10% weight loss)

Remember that these weight loss figures are distinct from the weight loss soon after birth. While 5% weight loss is common and within the normal range after birth, at any other time, weight loss is never normal. Clinical features of dehydration include decreased skin turgor, prolonged capillary refill time of more than two seconds, absent tears and dry mucous membranes, abnormal respiratory rate and pulse, tachycardia, sunken eyes and decreased urine output. However, the presence of just one of these signs is not thought to be strongly predictive of dehydration – more than one symptom would be considered necessary to make this diagnosis (Prisco et al, 2020). The search for the best clinical tool to assess dehydration continues (Falszewska et al, 2017). The NICE guideline does not recommend routine blood testing unless the child requires intravenous (IV) fluids, or if the child presents with clinical symptoms of shock or hypo/hypernatremia (NICE, 2009).

Sometimes children need an IV fluid bolus, and other times their dehydration can be managed orally. This will obviously be decided upon a case-by-case basis by the doctor in charge of the child's care. It's really important that if the child is too clinically unwell to breastfeed, or needs supplementing with formula, that the mother is helped and encouraged to maintain and perhaps if necessary, increase their milk supply, using many of the strategies that we reviewed in Chapter 7. Equally, if the child's weight has plateaued, or they have lost weight, the same suggestion applies. I have spoken to many mothers whose children have been admitted with diarrhoea and/or vomiting and subsequent dehydration and had NG feeds of formula despite an established milk supply. This occasionally happens when either the mother has also been unwell with the same infection and is clinically dehydrated and struggling to express. However, by far the most common reason for this scenario is failure to obtain a breast pump in a timely fashion. It is incredibly frustrating when there is clinical need for NG feeding, and the mother has a normal milk supply, but there is no practical way to get this down the NG tube. This is reason enough to have breast pumps located in the emergency department.

With weight loss, the exact cut-off point for intervention with supplementation will depend on the child's clinical condition. It will also depend on whether there are any risk factors indicated for that child that put them at greater risk, or mean that their individual level of tolerance is smaller.

Babies with hyperbilirubinaemia (jaundice) may need supplementation if they concurrently have weight loss or dehydration. Bilirubin binds to fat, so supplementing the baby with water is not a recommended strategy, as it will not support the excretion of bilirubin. Sometimes these babies need support not because their mother does not have enough milk, but because the baby is too sleepy to feed effectively. So once again, if the baby needs to be tube fed, we should still preferentially offer expressed milk first, unless this is unavailable.

Children who are fluid restricted for any reason often have a feeding plan that is worked out by the dietitian and paediatrician. Fluid restriction may occur with cardiac, renal, respiratory and other conditions. The difficulty with fluid restriction is that unmodified breastfeeding may be difficult, because it is very difficult to obtain the required number of calories with a reduced volume tolerance. This often means that the child needs to receive a high calorie formula so that the required number of calories can be delivered with a reduced total volume. It is often possible for *some* breastfeeding to occur, and this requires a sensitive conversation with the clinical team to ensure that breast milk is prioritised, alongside the restricted and high calorie fluids that the child requires. Having fluids restricted may not prevent the child from suckling on a well-drained breast for comfort. Depending on their clinical condition, it may be worth open-mindedly considering whether this is a possibility.

Other absolute reasons for supplementation include inborn errors of metabolism, such as galactosaemia and Phenylketonuria or PKU which I will return to in more detail later.

Finally, while children with hypoglycaemia do not categorically always require supplementation, if low blood sugars do not respond to optimal breastfeeding, or there is no expressed colostrum available to feed them, then this is another absolute indication for supplementation. Most guidelines suggest using formula, in this circumstance, like a medicine, using small amounts, and given via a cup or a spoon, while supporting and encouraging the mother to maintain or increase their milk supply as appropriate.

This is where it is important for practitioners unfamiliar with physiological milk volumes in breastfed babies and children to remind themselves of the consistency of milk volumes between 1-6 months. Asking mothers to produce 150ml/kg may not be either possible or indeed necessary for all mother-baby pairs. We will return to the key question of *how* to supplement a little later in the chapter.

Ensuring adequate milk intake

One of the main concerns for many health professionals is milk intake. Of course, the last thing anyone wants is for an infant to become dehydrated or for their weight to falter. In low-risk situations, usually low-tech means of assessment are sufficient – monitoring stool and urine output. This is especially reliable under six weeks – at least six heavy wet nappies and two to four soft yellow stools per day. After this time, stool output slows down due to the change in whey to casein ratio in the protein fraction of human milk.

In the hospital environment, daily weights may also be an option. But sometimes, it is necessary to ensure adequate weight gain or fluid volume from feed to feed, or conversely, in some conditions, ensure an infant does not drink too much.

One option is to use test weighing, with caution and compassion. Many years ago, test weighing was done frequently, and often unnecessarily, to objectify milk volumes ingested by infants. Many mothers from older generations can recall how this intervention spelled a lack of confidence and ultimately breastfeeding cessation in the 1970s. It can cause stress and pressure, which can inhibit the milk ejection reflex and therefore reduce the volumes ingested by the baby. However, when done skilfully, it can be a useful way to check weight and fluid volumes (Gregory, 2018). There remains controversy and disagreement over whether test weighing is accurate, and although research is patchy and often dated, in some studies, the data collected suggests a wide level of variance in accuracy (Savenije and Brand, 2006).

Test weighing should always be evaluated in a sensible way, remembering that a one-off test-weight is not necessarily reflective of all the other feeds across a 24-hour period. The test weights should also be evaluated in the context of an assessment of feeding efficiency and urine and stool output. You will also need very accurate scales – accurate to 2g or less, and you weigh the baby fully clothed before their feed. This is to keep them comfortable and minimise stress, crying and unnecessary additional tasks. Since we are only interested in the volume of milk, we can then weigh the baby after their feed without changing their nappy or clothes. Each 1g of weight gain is approximately equivalent to 1ml of milk drunk provided that the scales are accurate (Kent et al, 2015). Whether or not you decide to utilise test weights for a particular infant may depend on the resources available, what alternatives there are, and how accurate the measurement needs to be, as well as your clinical judgement.

How much to supplement?

There is not as much empirical evidence as you might imagine when it comes to how much supplement an infant should be offered. I'm grateful to Dr Ilana Levene for her exhaustive knowledge of fluid volume calculations and some of the sources of these recommendations. Many of the calculated fluid volumes are historic or based on formula-fed infants. They may not be suitable for breastfed babies who generally drink smaller volumes than bottle fed babies. A recent large systematic review found that breastfed babies drink approximately 7ml/kg/day on their first day of life, increasing to 69ml/kg/day by day 3. By two weeks of age, babies drink just over 150ml/kg/day. This volume then reduces steadily to around 107ml/kg/day by six months of age (Yeung, 2019). These volumes may differ for clinically unwell or unstable babies, those with higher calorie needs or large losses and secretions of course. But the standard paediatric fluid volume guidelines of 120ml/kg/day, 150ml/kg/day, or even 180ml/kg/day are probably inappropriate for all babies under two weeks of age, or over one month of age (i.e. most babies!).

Remember that there are many negative impacts of supplementing infants, so this should only be chosen as a strategy if it is genuinely medically indicated and essential. Supplementing infants can cause fluid overload in infants, negatively impact the mother's milk supply, expose the child to cows' milk protein (if formula is used), undermine maternal confidence, and lead to over-reliance on knowing the exact volume. This approach can make it harder for mothers to transition back to responsive, cue-led infant feeding. Many times, families have told me that they are advised to offer their baby a bottle at the end of a feed and 'see how much they will take'. This is a risky strategy if no anticipatory guidance is offered, such as how to pace the feed, how to simultaneously protect or increase the milk supply, or even the impact on milk supply that this may have. Gravity feeding a baby with a bottle to see what they will take is not a good way to decide how much milk the baby needs, especially without a fundamental understanding of how milk supply works. Babies have an instinctive suck reflex, and if they have a teat in their mouth, they will suck on it reflexively. If milk comes out, they will swallow it simply to protect their airway – it is neither a good test of hunger or milk deficit.

Finally, it is worth considering the risk of fluid overload for some babies. If breastfeeding is the physiological norm, then using formula volume calculations is arguably inappropriate, especially for children with some degree of compromise. While dehydration is certainly an issue of concern, overfeeding may also present challenges to sick infants and children. Sadly, this is an area that is not well-researched, though one study found that longer admission times were associated with higher levels of opiate sedation and more positive fluid balance, although this was not specific to breastfeeding (Mitting et al, 2021).

So, with the warnings and caveats about supplementation complete, and assuming that this supplement is medically necessary, you will need to come up with an approach to supplementing. This is best done in collaboration with the paediatric doctor in charge, the dietitian, a lactation advocate and of course, with the family being front and centre of all discussions.

Exactly how much supplement, and how important it is to know the volume, are clinical considerations, so the following are only suggestions and areas to consider, alongside your insider knowledge of the clinical situation you're trying to manage:

- Would it be possible to allow the infant to continue to breastfeed, and provide a supplement that the mother feels is suitable based on infant feeding cues? It's worth asking the question - do we actually *need* to know the volume? You don't necessarily have to provide a specific volume in all circumstances. Feeding to satiety can be an option for some children, provided that the infant is responsively fed. The danger with this approach is that if the infant is not being pace fed then they may drink beyond their hunger cues and overfeed. This is obviously detrimental to both confidence and milk supply. Some children with certain conditions may also struggle to regulate their appetite, rendering this approach less useful.

• Could you suggest a range of supplemental volume to offer instead of an exact amount? The range will clearly depend on how concerning their child's slow weight gain or clinical condition is, or how low the milk supply. For example, could you recommend offering between 30-60ml extra milk per feed, or 10-20ml, or 50-100ml? Having a range may feel less daunting, and offer some flexibility to allow the infant to decide how much they need, and acknowledge that appetite varies throughout the day, and indeed milk supply fluctuates throughout the day. Depending on the clinical circumstance, the volumes offered at each feed could be recorded if necessary, and the child could be weighed more frequently while the supplement is being given to easily and quickly identify if this strategy is working.

• What about suggesting a total additional volume to provide in a 24-hour period? This may work if the child does not need much supplementation and it is more manageable for the family to be able to decide when to offer the supplements per day. If, for instance, the total supplement needed is thought to be about 100ml per day, then the family may choose to offer this in multiple feeds with a syringe or cup, rather than disrupt breastfeeding and appetite regulation by offering a large volume via a bottle. On the other hand, the family may opt to give this all at once depending on what works for them.

• Have you thought about suggesting a *maximum* volume to offer? This may seem like a subtle language shift but suggesting to the family that they provide a *minimum* amount of milk may make them feel that they have to offer far more than that specified volume for fear of under-feeding their baby. However, if you suggest a maximum volume this may subtly suggest that providing more milk than that volume could compromise the milk supply and be unnecessary for the child's health and wellbeing.

- Be conscious of personal biases with supplements. We all have techniques we are most familiar and comfortable with and may default to recommending these. This is natural, but we should always remember that each child and family is unique. Not every baby with Prader Willi syndrome or a cardiac defect will need to be supplemented in the same way. Not every baby with a cardiac defect has a mother with a compromised milk supply. Not only are all children (even with the same condition) different, but they all have different mothers with different milk supplies. Try to be open minded and consider all the options with families.

- Consider too, who gives the supplement. Some mothers find it very emotionally difficult to provide a supplement to their child. If this is the case, it is important to not only praise and validate their efforts to breastfeed or provide breast milk, but also compassionately consider whether someone else could give this supplement to their baby. Some parents have told me that they have found it easier when their child had a nasogastric tube, because giving the formula down the tube felt more like a medical treatment, as opposed to a reflection of their inability to provide enough milk or calories. Other families found nasogastric tubes upsetting to look at and preferred a partner or nurse to bottle feed. Again, find out what is important to the family and where possible and clinically appropriate, try to be flexible.

Whichever approach the team and family decide is best for a specific baby, it is a good idea to think straight away about how you will support them to *get back* to exclusive or direct breastfeeding if this is desired, and possible. While not all families object to combination feeding, or continuing to express and supplement with expressed milk, this is very hard for some mothers. Try to offer suggestions for how to protect or increase milk supply at the same time as the supplement is required because time may be of the essence in terms of the capacity to produce more milk. Also consider a suggested time frame, so that the supplement is not perceived to be an ongoing strategy with no review or end-date. Provide a goal, and a date to review against that goal. Being specific is helpful; allowing families to plan for their baby's immediate future care.

Frequently needed specialist resources

Whenever babies cannot be directly breastfed, you will probably need equipment (unless the mother prefers to hand express, but you will still need a way to give the milk to the child). This may be simple equipment such as a pump, but it is likely that you will also need other tools, depending on parental preference and the clinical scenario.

While bottles are commonly thought to be the main way to supplement babies, there are many other options, such as nasogastric tubes, nipple shields, at-breast supplemental devices, and specialised bottles. Some children with complex feeding needs will require gastrostomy feeds, or total parenteral nutrition.

Feeding needs may change, develop, evolve over time, and also as the child's condition changes. Often a child will have many different approaches to managing their feeding, so the feeding tool in many cases should not be thought of as a fixed chapter in the child's feeding journey.

In reality, the child may transition from direct breastfeeding, to being nil by mouth, to nasogastric tube feeding, and then be rehabilitated back to the breast. Many children require some toggling back and forth between two or more different feeding methods as they adjust, get better, have bad days, or learn new skills. So, for a time, many children may be both directly breast-fed alongside receiving some nasogastric feeds or IV fluids. It's a good idea to prepare families for this, so that they aren't too disheartened if and when this happens or perceive it as a setback.

Each child and family will have a different feeding experience, diagnosis, response to illness, or specific challenges, and therefore it is impossible to say which babies will need which interventions. I will go through a variety of different feeding options, and the job of the feeding team will be to work out which is the most suitable. This is usually down to the feeding assessment, feeding goals and unique strengths, as well as challenges, of the child and family.

If the child has a complex condition, or the feeding has been very challenging, it is appropriate for a speech and language therapist, paediatrician, and dietitian to be involved alongside specialised lactation support. At the end of the chapter you will find a framework for decision making you can use within your MDT to help ensure that no part of the feeding journey is overlooked.

Paced bottle feeding

Bottles are probably the most common way to feed babies. Sometimes infants with orofacial anomalies such as cleft lip and palate are unable to directly breastfeed and need tools such as squeeze bottles or one way valve bottles because they cannot achieve the negative pressure required to effectively breastfeed (or indeed bottle feed from a standard bottle). Other times babies 'imprint' their suckling behaviours on a bottle, and struggle to effectively feed at the breast. This learned behaviour and muscle memory can sometimes mean that bottle feeding is the decision by default, sometimes after several attempts to get back to breastfeeding. For some families, for many different and valid reasons, the bottle could be reflective of parental choice.

Not so many years ago, there was an assumption that *everyone* knew how to bottle feed, but in the last 15-20 years there has been more research into feeding stress and how to minimise this. As professionals you may need to exercise some self-compassion and forgiveness here if this is the first time you have heard this. I have talked previously about the need for *'healthcare humility'* and the willingness to do things differently as a result of new information. I certainly remember as a nurse looking after infants on the ward who were being bottle fed and I cringe as I remember tapping on the bottle to coax the infant to finish their prescribed amount of milk. But, as Maya Angelou said; *'when we know better, we do better'.*

We now know that paced, responsive bottle feeding is less physiologically stressful, and provides a more nurturing feeding experience (Shaker, 2017). Ideally, we follow infant feeding cues, rather than feed on a fixed feeding schedule, and we do not force infants to finish their feed by tapping or twisting the bottle or coaxing the baby to drink more than they are showing they want to. If an infant cannot finish the minimum amount of feed which has been determined that they need, then they are probably not ready for full oral feeds. It's ok if there is a transition period between full tube feeding and full oral feeding.

During the bottle feed, hold the infant in as upright a position as possible (bearing in mind the comfort of the child with their condition), offering postural support if needed and allow frequent burp breaks. Maintain eye contact and observe for signs of feeding stress, which includes tightly shut eyes, colour change, clenched fists, or a splayed limb posture. Look out for facial grimace or frowning, a look of deep concentration, squirming, dribbling milk and/or the avoidance of eye contact. All these are probably signs of feeding stress and indicate that the baby needs a break.

Ideally, the infant should have a soft, relaxed posture, fists unclenched, eyes open and maintaining eye contact, and they should drink calmly with no gulping. A paced bottle feed should take at least 10-20 minutes, depending on the size of the feed.

Elevated side lying feeding

Another option for bottle feeding in infants who experience feeding stress is elevated side lying. They will need to have their head above the height of their hips, and it's usually more comfortable if the infant lies on their left side. Most caregivers place the infant on their lap, often on a pillow, and place their own feet on a footstool to lift their knees to facilitate the sloped position.

Compared with standard, semi-reclined feeding positions, elevated side lying feeding has been found to be less physiologically stressful for infants (Pados et al, 2017). You will still need to pause as needed, but many infants will manage a more coordinated suck-swallow-breathe sequence and fewer apnoeas in this position (Park et al, 2018).

At-breast supplementers

The supplemental at-breast tubes are becoming increasingly common for parents who wish to lactate for an adopted baby or want to restart lactation after a break. They are also good to prevent infants from imprinting on a bottle.

Essentially, with this method, a small tube is either taped near the nipple, or gently inserted into the baby's mouth during the feed and the baby receives their supplement at the breast. The other end of the tube is either placed inside a bottle of milk, or attached to a small container that can be worn around the mother's neck. It can be a good way of ensuring that the infant receives a required amount of milk, without exposing the baby to a different mechanism of sucking, which can make returning to direct exclusive breastfeeding harder. Babies receive all their milk at the breast, which means they associate the breast with food, and the mother also gets positive messages about their baby feeling satisfied and content at the breast which is also wonderful for bonding (Penny et al, 2018).

It can also help to transition a baby who has been bottle or tube fed back to breastfeeding, as the flow from the tube can be adjusted so that the infant gets a more rapid flow of milk to instantly reward them. Many mothers whose babies have never breastfed and become fussy or distressed at the breast, can use this technique to coax their babies back to the breast. Occasionally, if the baby has imprinted on a bottle or a nipple shield, the mother can wear a nipple shield while using the supplemental system, and often this will be a stepping stone to getting back to direct breastfeeding.

You can use expressed milk, donor milk, or formula, and in terms of products, there are a couple of commercial supplemental nursing systems, or you can make one using a five or six French nasogastric tube, with one end near the nipple, or in the baby's mouth, and the other end in a bottle of milk (Penny et al, 2019). As the baby gets more proficient at feeding, or as the milk supply increases, the amount of supplement can decrease, while monitoring the baby's weight gain.

The beauty of this device is that it can be used at home, so there is no need to wean from it prior to discharge. With most infants, the usual recommendation is to clean the tubing by flushing through with hot soapy water. With more vulnerable or at-risk infants another option is to use a sterile tube each time, though this is more resource heavy. Some units will recommend flushing the tube through with hot soapy water and then sterilising but local policies may vary.

Bridge device

Some families modify at-breast supplementers or use a nasogastric tube at the breast as a tool to get their infants to feed directly at the breast. There are in fact kits that comprise a nipple shield attached to a short tube with a large oral syringe. This enables the child to be fed at the breast, using either expressed breast milk or formula. The device is helpful for infants with a weak suck who would benefit from the increased sensory input from the firmer shield, or those who have developed a firm bottle preference. The kit was first developed by Kate Spivack IBCLC for her company Laally and has proven popular with mothers who have found the supplemental nursing systems fiddly. I am not aware of any clinical research with this device at the present time, and as with so many approaches to feeding in paediatrics, it may be a case of being open minded, creative and flexible in order to find a product that works for a particular child and family.

Nasogastric tubes

As with at-breast supplementers and bottles, nasogastric (NG) tubes can be used to feed expressed milk, donor milk or formula, and parents can and should be involved in NG feeding (Morag et al, 2019). NG feeds can happen while babies are being held skin to skin, or at a well-drained breast. This can also be a good way to help infants associate the breast with stomach fullness and satiety. Many babies will show some feeding behaviours at the breast when being NG fed, such as licking, nuzzling, rooting and even some suckling movements, which can be a good sign that an infant may be ready to try some direct feeding.

Sometimes babies who have a high calorie need, high metabolic load or who are sleepy or tire easily due to their condition can start off by feeding orally, and then have an NG feed. Other times it makes more sense to give a known amount of feed via the NG and then allow a baby who is fluid restricted to suckle on a well-drained breast to minimise fluid overload. Again, this should be a conversation between a combination of the parent, dietitian, paediatrician, paediatric infant feeding lead and speech and language therapist as appropriate to work out the best plan for an individual baby (Edwards et al, 2016).

Gastrostomy tubes

Percutaneous endoscopic gastrostomy (PEG) or 'G' tubes may be needed for infants and children with severe feeding difficulties as a more permanent way to manage calorie intake. They may also be tube fed due to problems such as unsafe swallow, or orofacial anatomical anomalies that make oral or NG feeding difficult. Other children who may need a G tube include those with higher metabolic load, for example children with congenital diaphragmatic hernia, cystic fibrosis, short gut and Pierre Robin sequence (Rosenberg et al, 2008; Rudra et al, 2016).

Children with G tubes often have them as a medium-term intervention, for example, after recovering from surgery, or they may be a longer-term feeding intervention. Many parents will be taught how to use overnight feeding pumps. Each child is different and will be under the care of a dietitian as well as the rest of the paediatric team.

While G tube feeding may feel very clinical for many families, there may be ways to make the feeding experience more nurturing, for example setting up and establishing positive, loving routines during feeding. These can include songs, reading stories, blowing bubbles, music, cuddling and holding during the feed, or even suckling at the breast in some cases.

Syringe feeding and finger feeding

Syringe and finger feeding are often not used as a long-term strategy, or indeed to feed large volumes. However, syringe or finger feeding can be a useful way of giving a small supplement, or helping a baby learn how to suckle. Parents do need to know how to aim the syringe into the baby's cheek, not straight into the mouth. Care is also needed not to squirt the milk forcefully as this risks aspiration. But a gentle pulse of milk in the side of the mouth of a baby who is not at risk of aspiration can work well.

Syringe feeding is particularly useful to give an additional bolus of high fat milk. This is often called *'hind-milk feeding'* in older textbooks. This is an old-fashioned term, since most of the lactation world reject the concept of foremilk and hindmilk, as the fat content of the feed gradually increases as the breast begins to be drained. That said, if it helps you understand the concept, that's ok. Mothers can be taught to hand express milk at the end of the feed to collect very high fat milk, and then offer this to their baby either in a syringe, or on a spoon. If the mother has an abundance of milk, or the infant is not able to drink all the milk their mother produces, you could leave the milk to stand and literally skim off the fat layer. This could be added to unmodified milk. Since about half the calories in milk are from the fat, even a small skim of cream added to milk could boost the calories by a significant amount. It can help to boost weight gain and maximise calorie intake, but of course, you will need to check with the dietitian and paediatrician to ensure that the child can tolerate the extra fat in their diet. This strategy also assumes an abundance of milk so it may not work for mothers who are struggling with their supply.

Finger feeding can encourage active suckling in some babies. The parent or clinician would place their finger, pad side towards the roof of the baby's mouth, about halfway along the baby's mouth, to stimulate a suckle. There can either be a syringe near the finger, or an NG tube, and the baby can be encouraged in this way to actively suckle while receiving a known volume of milk. There is some evidence to suggest that babies are more likely to return to full breastfeeding when they are finger fed, rather than bottle fed (Chantry et al, 2014).

Non-nutritive sucking

Non-nutritive sucking (NNS) can be a challenging concept for some professionals to get their heads around, unless you understand the value of breastfeeding beyond receiving milk. There are many reasons why non-nutritive sucking is clinically significant.

NNS can coax a child back to the breast, possibly alongside NG feeding. It can also be a way of providing mouth care. Even with very small amounts of human milk, the immunoglobulins present in milk can help line the gastrointestinal tract (Gephart et al, 2014). This may be particularly significant for immunocompromised children. Anecdotally, in my informal survey, several children receiving chemotherapy for various malignant diseases experienced no mucositis at all, including children undergoing bone marrow transplant.

NNS may help a child associate being near the breast with being full, and it is also well known that suckling reduces procedural pain (Harrison et al, 2016) and therefore this is a good way for mothers to provide comfort and reassurance to their child. Many mothers reported that breastfeeding helps them connect with their children during very stressful and worrying times. It is a 'normal' aspect of parenting and during seasons of many clinical interventions, parents highly value activities that feel normalising.

Finally, I've already mentioned that suckling a well-drained breast can be a good option for children whose fluid volume needs to be measured, without completely disrupting the feeding relationship. It is a way for mothers to connect with their children in a nurturing way and provide a safe space.

Getting back to the breast after ventilation/NG feeding

Whatever the reason for a feeding pause or disruption to feeding, it can sometimes be hard to get a little one back to the breast. I've heard many mothers at this point complain that they were not supported to make this final step and given dismissive responses such as *'it doesn't matter how they are fed as long as they are getting your milk'*. This isn't true. Pumping is not without effort, and if a mother wishes to return to direct breastfeeding this is important. It's often much easier to feed a baby directly than continue to pump and bottle feed. How to get back to direct feeding depends on the unique situation of the family, and a feeding assessment is required to create a bespoke plan.

Broadly though, after suctioning, ET tube placement, CPAP or tube feeding, some infants need some time and patience to get back to breastfeeding. It may be because they have associations with unpleasant experiences or sensations in their mouth or throat, or because they are essentially out of practice at oral feeding. Sometimes a baby needs to be gently worked up towards full oral feeds again. Other children experience withdrawal after prolonged use of opiate-based pain relief, and others have iatrogenic vocal cord palsy, neurological trauma/injury or complications resulting in impaired reflexes.

When supplements and feeding pauses are medically necessary.

One mother of a child with a complex medical history coped relatively well with a plethora of setbacks and difficulties, but their breastfeeding journey nearly came to an abrupt and unwanted end after an admission with bronchiolitis.

"After his liver transplant, Lewis carried on breastfeeding well until a severe case of RSV positive bronchiolitis resulted in a PICU admission where he was ventilated for nine days. When he was extubated, he refused to breastfeed and his mother, Anna, was devastated. She worked closely with the dietitian, speech and language therapist and paediatrician and they carefully reduced the NG feeds to help Lewis develop his appetite. Alongside this, Anna continued to have skin to skin with Lewis, continued expressing, tried to stay calm (not easy!) and patiently waited for him to be ready. After a 2-day nursing strike, he went back to the breast."

I've known many babies seemingly go on a 'nursing strike' upon recovery or extubation. It's obviously very worrying and distressing for parents when this happens, but some gentle handling and calm is often required here. It's a good idea to dim the lights, use quiet voices, and remain very calm. A mother can try skin-to-skin, or babywearing.

A good option is to finish at the breast so that the child associates the breast with satiety, comfort and calm rather than at the beginning of the feed when they may be hungrier and more frantic, especially if the flow rate from the breast is slow. *'Finish at the breast'* is a strategy coined by Dr. Christina Smillie, who has found it to be more successful than starting on the breast. She points out that if babies are really hungry, and the flow rate from the breast is slow (especially if the pressure is high and the mother is stressed), the baby is likely to fuss and become frustrated. This in turn undermines parental confidence. Due to this being a stressful situation, mothers will often end up aborting the feed attempt and giving a bottle. The more this happens, the more detrimental the impact on milk supply. By starting on the bottle, the baby can have their acute hunger satiated, and then go to the breast feeling less ravenous. With a calmer feed, the mother is more likely to relax, the baby is more likely to feed effectively, and the milk supply is therefore more likely to be maintained.

Another good hack is to feed the baby when they are sleepy, just waking from a nap, or consider bed sharing to take advantage of sleepier lying-down feeds. Babies will sometimes instinctively or reflexively suckle in light sleep, which can coax them back to feeding. This is especially useful for older babies who often demonstrate their preference very vocally!

If the child has become accustomed to a bottle teat, sometimes a thin silicone nipple shield can coax a baby back to the breast. Basically, making the breast feel like the familiar silicone can help a baby accept the breast. While it is not the same as direct breastfeeding, it at least removes the need to pump and bottle feed, thus making the feeding more efficient. Babies do sometimes imprint on a certain type of teat/nipple, especially if it was introduced in the first few days (Wambach and Spencer, 2019), so it can be harder to get a baby to accept feeding from a bare breast. The nipple shield can act as a conduit to that goal. The Laally bridge may also assist with these situations.

Another option is to form the thumb and forefinger into a 'U' shape and cup the breast from underneath, then push the hand back towards the chest wall. This will firm up the breast tissue. Sometimes it is the firm feeling of a teat that babies have become accustomed to, and therefore making the breast tissue feel tighter and firmer can smooth the transition. This can also be a good way of easing a baby away from a nipple shield. Other mothers try the *'bait and switch'* approach – starting on the nipple shield or bottle, and after a few minutes, quickly removing it and seeing if the baby will latch. In my experience, a lot of patience and perseverance is required, but I have known babies come back to the breast after bottle feeding or using a nipple shield for 3-4 months or more.

While waiting for a baby to be ready, some mothers also try to make bottle feeding more like breastfeeding. While this statement is slightly oxymoronic, there are ways to make bottle feeding feel like a bridge back to breastfeeding. For example, babies can be bottle fed skin to skin, or cheek to breast. If both parents have been feeding the baby, the mother can take over full responsibility for feeds, to help the baby associate their mother with feeding. Parents can slow the flow rate from the bottle, either by using a slower teat, or allowing the baby to suckle on an empty teat for a minute before allowing milk to flow, so that the baby gets used to a flow rate that is not instantaneous. This is where skilled paced bottle feeding can be so helpful, allowing breaks and pauses to mimic the variable flow rate from the breast.

Milk flow rates that are slow, can, as I said, make feeding more difficult for a baby who is used to the rapid and consistent flow from a bottle. Reducing stress and tension for the family, along with privacy and lots of encouragement will minimise stage fright and an inhibited milk ejection reflex.

Finally, babies are more likely to actively feed and stay on the breast if there is milk flowing. Using breast compressions to increase the flow rate of milk can help. This is a simple and low-tech way of making feeding more efficient and can also help a sleepy baby. To effectively breast compress, the mother simply gets a big handful of breast tissue and gently squeezes and holds for a couple of seconds. You would then observe the baby to monitor active swallowing during this intervention. It's important to release the pressure between compressions, to prevent blocked ducts, but the mother can continue to breast compress for the duration of the feed if they need to. In practice, I have found this useful for babies who are sleepy, or who quickly lose interest in feeding, as well as those who need to maximise calorie intake with the minimum amount of energy expenditure.

Children experiencing iatrogenic withdrawal

When children are critically unwell in PICU, sedating analgesia is a common and necessary intervention to reduce pain and suffering, as well as to prevent them from moving and accidentally displacing endotracheal tubes, drains and central lines. The medications usually chosen are opioids and benzodiazepines although different units may have different protocols. In general, the longer a child is exposed to these sedating analgesics, the more likely they are to experience withdrawal, although tolerance obviously varies. Symptoms of withdrawal include tachypnoea (rapid breathing), nausea and vomiting, sweating, hypertonia and irritability (Ávila-Alzate et al, 2020). Withdrawal has been found to be under-reported and under-treated, and furthermore, unvalidated or inappropriate scales are sometimes used to measure withdrawal. For example, some units use the neonatal withdrawal scale, which means that mothers are sometimes subjected to unnecessary questions about *their* opioid use, rather than more accurate questions about *their child's* opiate exposure.

While weaning a child off sedating analgesics is not an exact science, many approaches have been proposed (Sneyers et al, 2020) which are not within the scope of this book to discuss. What is important to note here is that parents could be better prepared for some of the possible behaviours that their opiate exposed child might exhibit after extubation and/or weaning from analgesia. Preparation for the behaviour changes is important as iatrogenic withdrawal might affect the child's breastfeeding behaviour. Many mothers have anecdotally reported that their child wanted to breastfeed non-stop or was extremely irritable. This is demoralising, and requires great compassion and additional support, as well as practical strategies. Some children settle better when held in skin-to-skin contact, while others seem to prefer less handling. Some children are thirsty, so rather than feeding round the clock, they might settle with water if this is clinically appropriate. Other mothers choose to offer small amounts of additional formula in these situations, as a temporary measure.

When feeding needs to be paused

There are sometimes circumstances where feeding needs to be paused, as opposed to the child being supplemented, which I will now briefly discuss. Some conditions are rare, and yet I mention them because they have previously been major barriers to maintaining breastfeeding, such as phenylketonuria (PKU), and chylothorax. The other reason for specifically mentioning these rare conditions is that while they may be rare on a population level, if a professional is working in a highly specialised tertiary referral hospital, then several of those babies may be seen in one unit disproportionately, making it a much more significant clinical problem to address. After all, the fact that a problem is rare is meaningless if you are the one parent whose child happens to have that condition. Other situations are far more common, for example pre-operative fasting, respiratory support and severe illness.

Fasting times

There are no nationally agreed guidelines for fasting, and local policies may vary. The Academy of Breastfeeding Medicine suggests four hours nil by mouth prior to surgery for breast fed babies, and six hours for formula fed babies (ABM, 2012). Infants can have clear fluid an hour before.

However, gastric emptying times have been found to be far less than six hours, even for exclusively formula fed infants (Bonner et al, 2015). Generally, it is found in many studies that the speed of gastric emptying is faster with larger volumes as well. Given how distressing it is both for infants and mothers to withhold feeding, this is perhaps an area that needs urgent evaluation.

A recent meta-analysis found that gastric half emptying time is 57 minutes on average (Beck et al, 2019), which makes a four-hour pre-operative fast seem fairly draconian. Nevertheless, it sometimes takes time to see shifts in policy and procedures, and in the meantime, you will probably have to support parents who are trying to soothe their distressed and hungry infants or toddlers, as well as maintain their milk supply. It is often helpful to involve a support person who isn't lactating, so that the baby cannot smell leaking milk. Carrying infants, rocking or swaying, or distracting them with play if age-appropriate can all help get through this common, but frustrating scenario. Another difficult scenario for some mothers is when they are tandem feeding two children, and one is nil by mouth and the other is not. This may require some support from the play team, or a partner to distract the nil-by-mouth child while the other child is given a feed out of sight.

Many babies and children can breastfeed once they have recovered from their anaesthetic, depending on their stability and clinical condition, and both mothers and children may find this comforting and a good way to reconnect after the stress of surgery and separation.

One practical consideration is to remember that some children may be nauseous after a general anaesthetic. Depending on the age, cognition and condition of the child, it may be pragmatic to offer the child some sips of water to see if this is tolerated first or offer the child a well-drained breast. Many parents find that if their child has multiple anaesthetics, they develop insight into how their child usually responds and know if their child is usually prone to vomiting. Antiemetic medications may be appropriate for some children.

Sometimes children who have been fasted for a considerable length of time (whether due to the length of time in surgery, or a delayed procedure) sometimes want to guzzle. For some children, these large feeds are well tolerated, while for others, a large volume of milk in an empty stomach can sometimes make them vomit. This can't always be prevented if it is the first or a one-off occasion, but parents are usually very good historians and will have insight into whether their child has a tendency to do this if they have had repeat procedures. One option if they are known to vomit easily is to suggest that the mother express some milk prior to offering their child a feed, to reduce the volume and flow rate.

Finally, if the surgery/procedure is delayed, or the child is under anaesthetic for a long time, the mother may become uncomfortable. This depends hugely on the age of the child, the breast storage capacity and individual responses to stress and missed feeds. Some mothers have told me that they did not experience any discomfort, as their child was older and only feeding minimally. Others have reported that they became painfully full and suffered blocked ducts. Having proactive conversations prior to surgery to make a simple plan for managing this is a sensible idea.

Illness, instability and incompatibility

Another common scenario is the baby who is too unwell to orally feed. For most admissions, this will be relatively short in duration, though as I've already said, these acute and self-limiting conditions are associated with a high rate of breastfeeding disruption, so should be treated carefully. If breastfeeding must be paused so that the child can receive intensive care, surgery or respiratory support for example, then the golden rule is to protect the milk supply, usually by expressing. If the baby can tolerate the milk, the expressed milk can be tube fed, used for oral trophic feeds, mouth care or saved for when the baby recovers. Sometimes a critically sick child will not be able to handle their usual volume of milk, but they may be able to be fed a small quantity via their enteral feeding tube. Sometimes mothers report this as a blessing in disguise because the stress of their child being so ill sometimes has a profound effect on their milk ejection reflex and ability to pump their usual volumes of milk. If there *is* a surplus of milk, then this can be stored.

One word of caution here – I have heard many mothers tell me that they were told that their milk was filling up the freezer or taking up too much space. On the face of it, this is a reasonable and practical issue that needs to be addressed. However, it needs to be handled very sensitively, because they may interpret this as meaning they or their milk are a burden, or getting in the way. This is especially relevant as parents of critically sick children may already be at risk of feeling like a spare part and uninvolved. It is essential that we value the milk they are producing and handle the storage issue with tact and compassion.

Some children with respiratory compromise can continue to breastfeed to some extent, while they are carefully observed to ensure that they do not become compromised by their increased work of breathing. Some children end up pulling on and off the breast or turning a lighter colour when they have respiratory distress – which is sometimes the first sign of their respiratory compromise that parents are aware of. This may in turn cause several outcomes:

- Frustration for the mother and child
- Nipple soreness
- Inadequate milk intake
- Oxygen desaturation
- Fullness and engorgement

For these reasons, careful observation of a feed is essential to assess whether the child is a) removing milk effectively enough, and b) not becoming unstable. If it is established that the child cannot feed effectively due to their current condition, a careful plan must be established to treat the child's condition and maintain an appropriate amount of milk via an alternative route, as well as to protect the milk supply.

There is variation in practice regarding continuing oral feeds while on non-invasive respiratory support such as CPAP and high flow nasal cannula (HFNC) oxygen. Once again, there is far more literature relating to the preterm population than the paediatric population, and one paper found that continuing oral feeding was more prevalent in NICU than PICU (Canning et al, 2020). Some of the concerns relate to fears over whether the continuous flow of oxygen may interfere with the coordination of breathing and thus inadvertently cause aspiration – which can occur without obvious signs and symptoms such as choking or coughing (Dumpa et al, 2020).

This is where working with speech and language therapists (SLTs) is imperative. Any child who is at risk of airway compromise should be reviewed with the SLT team, who are highly experienced at assessing and managing swallowing and breathing in medically complex children.

Less common reasons for pausing breastfeeding include infants with inborn errors of metabolism, including PKU. Many years ago, these infants were put on Phe free formula, but current best practice is to encourage breastfeeding, titrated against blood Phe levels, since infant cognitive outcomes are optimised (Riva et al, 1996).

Chylothorax is even more unusual, and yet, for the small number of mothers facing this challenge with their children every year, mostly in cardiac units, it can be a significant barrier to maintaining breastfeeding. Chylothorax is a rare condition that can be associated with a number of congenital conditions including Noonan's syndrome, Down syndrome/Trisomy 21, and Tracheoesophageal Fistula, but about 65% of all cases are associated with conditions that necessitate chest surgery. Surgical chylothorax is a rare but known complication of major cardiac surgery. It involves an accumulation of chyle (which is a mix of fat, protein and immunological components including immunoglobulins) in the pleural space. Loss of chyle to the pleural space can result in malnutrition and increased risk of infection (Haines et al, 2014).

Traditional treatments include surgical intervention, with an indwelling chest drain, stopping all enteral feeds and moving to total parenteral nutrition, using IV octreotide – which blocks lymph flow in the thoracic duct, or moving to a medium chain triglyceride diet instead of long chain fatty acids (Bui et al, 2019). Since human milk fat is long chain fatty acid based, this has historically meant pausing or stopping breastfeeding, usually for several weeks. Medium chain triglycerides, or MCTs, are absorbed into the venous rather than lymphatic system, and so dietary modification can manage the condition.

However, this means stopping breastfeeding, and either pumping and storing/donating milk, usually for about six weeks - or stopping altogether. There is also the concern that human milk contains immunoglobulins which would be particularly significant for babies with serious conditions, who are at higher risk of infection.

There are no national guidelines, and local policies vary enormously both nationally and internationally. Several paediatric centres around the world have developed a policy of defatting human milk and giving fortified skimmed milk to babies. Skimmed milk has half the number of calories, so MCTs, vitamins and sometimes MCT formula is added, but it means that infants still receive the protection of immune factors in their mother's milk. A small number of studies have explored the feasibility of this and found that growth rates were sufficient when the milk was fortified (Concheiro-Guison et al, 2019).

To skim the milk, this can either be carried out by refrigerated centrifugation, or a low-tech option is to simply allow the milk to separate and skim off the fat, involving the dietitian to monitor growth and nutritional requirements.

With all these complex issues, the bottom line is that this is about valuing human milk as a living fluid that doesn't just provide nutrients, but important immunological components, and also - perhaps equally importantly - it is a way of parenting and mothering. Creatively thinking of ways to continue breastfeeding to provide human milk, sends a powerful message to parents about how important they are, how involved they can be, and how significant some of the non-medical things they can do for their child are.

A multi-disciplinary decision-making framework for breastfed children on the paediatric ward

It often helps to have a structured approach to considering all the options when you are working with a child with medical complexity. This is my assessment process that I have used to support children with illnesses and conditions:

Child's name
Mother and significant family members names
Child's age
Child's feeding status prior to admission (exclusive BF/combination fed/tube feeding/solids)
What are the mother's feeding goals?
Child's condition
Is this condition acute or chronic? (i.e. is this disruption to feeding likely to be recurring?)
Is there a specific clinical concern or complication at this time? (e.g.. respiratory distress, dehydration, aspiration)
Expected duration of admission
Is it likely that long-term adaptations to breastfeeding will have to be made?
What is this child's specific breastfeeding challenge? (e.g. difficult positioning, low tone, fluid restriction)
Does the mother have any breastfeeding concerns? (e.g. nipple pain, breast infection)
Has a breastfeeding assessment been undertaken?
Are there any concerns about milk production or intake? (e.g. ineffective feeding, fatigue causing insufficient milk transfer, low milk supply, hyperlactation, forceful MER)
Are they clinically stable enough to attempt direct breastfeeding?
Are there relevant necessary clinical interventions that are barriers to direct breastfeeding? (e.g. oxygen therapy, strict fluid balance, minimal handling)

Are these restrictions on direct breastfeeding justified? (i.e. could a flexible compromise be found?)
Do I need to involve any other specialists? (e.g. SLT, dietitian, lactation specialist, paediatrician)
Does this mother require any practical or emotional strategies or support? (e.g. counsellor, food, financial assistance, transport)
What breastfeeding adaptations could we try?
If this child requires supplementation, what is the most suitable method? (consider donor human milk if available, cup, NG, at-breast supplementation, bridge device etc)
If breastfeeding needs to be paused, what strategies have been promoted to protect the maternal milk supply?
What responsive activities could be suggested to protect the parent-child bond during this admission? (e.g. bedsharing, skin to skin, carrying, containment holding)
Suggested plan, co-created with family and relevant professionals
Date for review

© Lyndsey Hookway

Test yourself:

1. Which of the following is NOT a medically necessary reason to supplement?

   a. Baby with Down's Syndrome.

   b. Clinically significant dehydration.

   c. Hypoglycaemia that is unresponsive to optimised breastfeeding.

   d. Phenylketonuria.

2. Which of the following is a sensible reason to consider test weighing?

   a. When babies are fluid restricted.

   b. When babies are transitioning from tube to oral feeds.

   c. To reassure parents that their baby is feeding well.

   d. All the above.

3. Which of the following methods of feeding is least likely to interfere with an infant's ability to breastfeed?

   a. Syringe feeding.

   b. Paced bottle feeding.

   c. At-breast supplementer.

   d. Nasogastric tube feeding.

4. Regarding preoperative fasting times, which of the following is correct?

   a. Human milk has a slightly faster gastric emptying time than formula.

   b. There are national guidelines supporting the 4-hour pre-operative fasting rationale.

   c. Local policies regarding fasting times may vary.

   d. Both a and c are correct.

Chapter 9

Supporting feeding in specific circumstances

No matter how complex the situation, if you remember the three golden rules with feeding support, you won't go far wrong. **Keep the baby fed** (preferably with the mother's own milk), **protect the milk supply**, and **manage the existing problem** so that the baby can return to their usual way of feeding as quickly and as safely as possible. As I have said a few times, my **additional** recommendation is to consider how to compensate for the lack of closeness and skin contact that is inevitable with feeding interruptions.

For some conditions, you may need to draw on some specific tools and supportive feeding strategies to manage feeding, which I will share with you. I would also urge everyone to not assume that a baby will be unable to feed based solely on their experience of previous babies with the same condition. This is where the individual feeding assessment is so important. Allow babies and children to surprise you!

Involving the MDT may also be important for babies who are not coping with feeding despite good feeding support. Remember that poor feeding can be diagnostically significant, and it is often the first sign that an infant is sick or compensating. There may also be an evolving problem that has yet to be diagnosed. So, whether the infant has an acute or chronic condition, whatever the underlying cause of their medical problem, if there are feeding challenges, the parents are concerned, or you cannot explain what is going on, refer on. It's always good when we can put our finger directly on something, but sometimes the cause takes some detective work, and feeding difficulty may be the first clue, so trust your gut instinct and involve senior colleagues.

There is clearly a need to stay in your sphere of competence here, so remember to use the multidisciplinary team, and refer to more experienced colleagues – either clinical or lactation professionals when you need to.

Acute illness

The most common reason for admission is acute illness. You already know from the Heilbronner study (2017) that a brief stay in hospital can negatively impact breastfeeding. For this reason, it is a good idea to make feeding assessments mandatory for all infants under the age of one, and older children where appropriate, even when the expected length of stay is just one to three days.

Many of you in the paediatric setting know this, but for our lactation and non-medical colleagues, it is worth remembering that 'acute' does not necessarily mean 'minor' or not serious. Children can be extremely unwell for a short length of time, can deteriorate rapidly, or become suddenly unwell with little to no warning. Always remember that acute illness can be shocking and traumatic for families.

With acute illness, the clinical priority will be to stabilise the child and treat their condition, but alongside that, we also need to be thinking about the milk that the child will need once they are well enough again. Often, sick children do not feel well enough to feed, are fatigued, or do not finish a feed. Acute problems for the mother include engorgement, which will downregulate milk supply quickly, and blocked ducts. It is therefore important to remember that in protecting a milk supply we are not only safeguarding the child's milk for they are well enough to feed, but also preventing the mother from becoming unwell or uncomfortable and protecting her mental health and parenting self-efficacy. We cannot simply pause milk production during a period of acute illness, and then restart once a child is better. We need to actively protect it.

The mother may need lots of support to get around problems of stage fright and pressure to pump, especially if she is stressed and anxious about their child's condition. While mothers absolutely have the right to pump wherever they prefer to, they may desire to be given some privacy, so always offer a screen to enable cot or bedside pumping. Health professionals are used to seeing people in various states of undress, but some mothers are more reserved or have religious privacy preferences. While it may not bother us to walk in on a mother who is hand expressing or pumping, it may embarrass or intimidate the mother. Also, using a pump is very different to breastfeeding. While some mothers have no qualms about breastfeeding in public, they may feel differently about expressing in front of others - don't assume that a mother who is happy to breastfeed in public feels the same about the pump. Remember to be respectful of differing viewpoints regarding this personal issue, and offer them a choice of places to pump, as well as remembering to alert the parent with a verbal or visual clue that you are approaching or about to pull back the curtain so that they can cover up if they prefer to.

Another closely related issue is one of 'enforced privacy'. Many mothers have told me that health professionals drew curtains or screens around them while they were breastfeeding on an open ward, without being asked to. This can make them feel like they are doing something 'dirty' or shameful and many mothers have described this behaviour to me with considerable anger and frustration. Privacy should be *offered*, not enforced or assumed. Not all mothers are bothered by feeding in public. Furthermore, many mothers have told me that they were waiting to hear results of tests or procedures and when the healthcare professional came to report their findings or tell them what the plan was, and saw that they were breastfeeding, they turned around and left. This will delay them from receiving information about their child. There is often no need to do this. Many mothers would rather the professional remained present to give their information, than delay it. The bottom line is to ask, rather than assume either way.

You will probably need to draw on the counselling skills and distraction techniques we covered in Chapter 7. We should also not be jumping straight to supplements of formula but encouraging mothers to express and valuing the milk that they are already producing, as well as the comfort that breastfeeding brings to an acutely unwell child. Siting cannulas and taking blood can be done while a child is nursing, it provides pain relief, and nebulisers or oxygen can be given while a child is held close to a parent. Children who need additional support will still benefit from skin to skin and breastfeeding in many cases. Also, where possible, try to avoid being prescriptive about the regularity of feeds. Strict three or four hourly feeding routines are not evidence-based. If there are concerns about hydration status then children's intake can be monitored in other ways other than measured NG or bottle feeds – for example monitoring nappy output, daily weights, or pre and post feed weights if there is enough concern.

If a child cannot orally feed without significant compromise, then nasogastric feeding has been shown to be preferable over IV fluids and importantly, is less painful and better tolerated (Oakley et al, 2013).

Providing supplemental oxygen and suctioning has also been shown to support children to continue to orally feed during acute respiratory infections (Karampatsas et al, 2019; Griffiths et al, 2020; NICE, 2015; 2021)

Some helpful practical suggestions for children with respiratory distress who are clinically stable enough to orally feed include:

- Upright feeding, with the child straddling one leg either side of the mother's thigh.
- Shorter, more frequent feeds, as the child may be better at tolerating a) smaller volumes and b) shorter bursts of active feeding with an opportunity to rest in between.
- Breast compressions may decrease the effort a child has to make in order to feed.
- Wafting oxygen to combat the slight desaturation during feeding has been found to be helpful for children who do not require HFNC oxygen or CPAP.

Hypotonia (low tone)

There are many conditions that may mean that a child has low muscle tone. Most of the available literature at this time refers to children with Down's syndrome, but there are many other conditions that may cause a baby to have low tone.

Hypotonia makes feeding difficult because children often have less control of their neck muscles, causing their head to lag. They also tend to struggle because they have low tone in their limbs, so cannot use their arms and legs for positional and stabilising support at the breast (Walker, 2008). They also may have poor tone in the muscles that are less obvious – such as their cheeks, tongue and face.

Children with low tone often need some positional and postural support for feeding. Upright or koala hold feeding can be helpful. The baby will sit on their mother's lap, with their legs straddling their mother's thigh, and the mother can use their arms to support their baby's head. If the mother leans back slightly, gravity will help to pull the child closer towards them, offering more feeding stability and allowing the infant's tongue to drop down and forward (Thomas et al, 2016).

To stimulate a gape, you can touch the middle of their lower lip, which should make them open their mouth, and they may need head and neck support unlike most children who are not hypotonic.

Dancer hand support is a well-established lactation technique that provides stability to the baby's jaw and weak masseter muscles. The mother's hand is positioned under their breast and moves forward so that the three smallest fingers support underneath the breast. The index finger and thumb then form a U shape and are positioned on either side of the baby's face, applying gentle pressure to the cheeks to stabilise them, and keep the baby on the breast (Wambach and Spencer, 2019).

Another tool that may help is a thin silicone nipple shield, which may offer more stability in the infants' mouth and provide greater sucking stimulation, particularly if the baby has under-developed buccal pads or weak masseter muscles.

Higher calorie need

For children with some conditions, there may be increased energy requirements of 30-50% which cannot always be met with exclusive breastfeeding (Wambach and Spencer, 2019). If the condition is known antenatally, some mothers have been known to deliberately induce an oversupply from the beginning, imagining that they are pumping for twins. Some children need all this extra milk, while others may have high calorie needs and *also* be fluid restricted. In these cases, with some of the excess milk they produce, they can allow the milk to separate and reserve the cream layer, which they use to supplement their expressed milk that has not been separated (Mangel et al, 2015). Strategies such as this obviously are not appropriate for all children, and should be worked out with dietetic and paediatric involvement

Sometimes, particularly if some of the fatty fraction of milk is given to supplement regular pumped milk, mothers can avoid the need for supplementation, as one mother in my informal survey managed to do with her child who was diagnosed antenatally with hypoplastic left heart syndrome. But this requires an investment in time and knowledge at the very beginning of lactation, as well as high levels of commitment from the mother. In many cases, even with all the preparation possible, a mother will not be able to make enough milk to meet their child's calorie requirement, so this is far from being a universally recommended strategy.

For children whose condition is not known until after lactation is established, it may be far harder to increase milk supply to meet the additional calorie needs that are caused by the child's condition. As well as cardiac conditions, other examples include cystic fibrosis and certain gut related problems.

For babies with who need additional calories, some strategies such as breast compressions, more frequent feeding and fat-rich top ups of hand expressed milk may help, but supplements, or fortification may be required to maintain optimal growth.

Other children whose calorie or fluid needs may exceed realistic breast milk output include children with high outputs either from secretions, stoma losses or diarrhoea and vomiting. In these cases, it is sometimes simply not possible to replace all the fluids lost, and children may need additional fluids and milk.

This situation requires a great deal of tact and compassion, as it's easy for mothers to feel like their milk is 'not good enough'. I find it is helpful to remind them firstly of all the immunological support they continue to offer their children through their milk, but also to help them imagine that *their* milk is exclusively feeding their baby. The supplement is essentially feeding their child's condition or replacing fluid losses. Some mothers find a great deal of comfort from separating it out and thinking of the supplement as 'medicine' or 'fluid replacement'.

It's really important that these issues are addressed with the MDT, as dietetic support is really important particularly in more complex cases where a child has high calorie needs but is also fluid restricted. Managing their energy, micronutrients, mineral and fluid needs can be very challenging, so work with your colleagues to come up with creative solutions. This may involve some trial and error. I have spoken to several mothers who have worked with a supportive dietitian who has reviewed the child's weight on a regular basis to finesse the feeding plan in order that the mother's feelings and wishes, as well as the child's nutritional and calorie needs were prioritised.

Do babies get tired at the breast?

I briefly touched on this subject during the explanation of how breastfeeding works, but it is worth digging into something that I hear a lot of health professionals saying to parents. Many mothers are told that if an infant is at the breast for longer than a certain arbitrary amount of time, often around 20 minutes, they will get tired. Most of the time, we are looking at this in the wrong way. Comfort suckling, and being at the breast is not a problem per se.

In a healthy baby who is effectively transferring milk, being at the breast for any length of time for non-nutritive suckling in addition to nutritive suckling is not going to waste calories, in the same way that suckling on a dummy or pacifier doesn't waste calories for those children.

There are two main issues that we *do* need to consider though. The first one is that some babies may spend a long time at the breast but are not actually feeding effectively. If this happens, professionals who are not assessing for milk transfer may be falsely reassured by a long feed, assuming that plenty of milk has been taken in – equating the length of feed with the volume ingested.

The other issue is that some babies with low tone, high calorie need, sleepy babies, sick babies, preterm or neurologically impaired babies may become fatigued *before* they have actually consumed enough milk. These babies may fall asleep before they have actually had enough milk. This obviously presents a risk to the child, but also to the milk supply. While milk supplies can be built back up or even induced from no supply at all, this is obviously much more work.

We need to remember that some babies may be significantly compromised and may have to work much harder to remove milk. They may tire not necessarily from feeding, but the muscle control and maintaining alertness that feeding requires. It's also important to remember that feeding does cause a degree of physiological stress even in healthy babies, and for a compromised infant, that additional stress may be too much. However, we need to position this in context. The assumption is often that breastfeeding is too tiring, but evidence has demonstrated that bottle feeding is more physiologically stressful. Arguably, if an infant would find breastfeeding too tiring, they will find all oral feeding too tiring, though of course all children are different. It is important that we are careful about the subtle and not so subtle messages that mothers hear when we suggest the blanket approach that breastfeeding is tiring.

Provided that those children are supported to feed effectively or are fed in a way that ensures they have enough volume and calories, there is no reason why they cannot comfort suckle as well. This may serve to protect the nurturing act of breastfeeding that can be lost with alternative methods of supplementation.

Metabolic diseases

Several metabolic diseases are currently tested for on the newborn blood spot, alongside conditions such as congenital hypothyroidism and cystic fibrosis. Not all are tested for in the newborn period and therefore some present in later infancy. One of the metabolic errors is Phenylketonuria, or PKU. PKU is a recessive inherited disorder that leads to a defect in the enzyme phenylalanine hydroxylase which prevents the proper metabolism of phenylalanine, or Phe. This defect causes Phe to build up in the brain and tissues. To prevent brain damage, the amount of Phe must be limited, starting in the first month of life.

The levels of Phe in human milk are far lower than the levels in regular formula and the amount of Phe decreases over time, so most mothers are encouraged to continue to breastfeed alongside regular blood tests. The mothers then have to adjust how much they are able to breastfeed and how much Phe-free formula they need to give. In a retrospective cohort study, children with PKU who were breastfed alongside their Phe free formula from infancy had a 12.9 IQ point advantage over children exclusively fed Phe free formula, after adjusting for socioeconomic differences and maternal educational level which may be a motivating factor (Riva et al, 1996). Greve et al (1994) developed a protocol to calculate how much Phe free formula the child needs to keep their Phe at the required level.

Galactosaemia is a rare recessive inherited trait that causes the deficiency of one of the enzymes needed for lactose metabolism. With this condition, any consumption of galactose results in multiorgan dysfunction and infants are at risk for severe illness including cognitive impairment and liver disease. They usually present in the first few days of life with diarrhoea and vomiting, poor weight gain and lethargy. If the child is found to have one of the variant forms, some breastfeeding in combination with lactose-free formula may be possible.

Both conditions will require coordinated care between the dietitian, paediatrician and lactation specialist. Mothers who are not able to exclusively breastfeed need lots of support to maintain their milk supply. You might imagine that if they only need a partial milk supply that this would be easier to do, but constantly having to juggle how much feeding they can do according to blood results is difficult and stressful, and there is a psychological impact that needs to be considered. Imagine how hard it is to manage the emotional aspect of knowing that if you were to exclusively breastfeed, your baby could be neurologically impaired. Balancing the need to manage their condition, alongside compromising on their intended feeding goals isn't easy.

Mothers need to be able to deal with the grief of not being able to exclusively breastfeed, while also juggling the extra workload of partial breastfeeding, and regular testing. It's important to stress to parents the advantages of continuing to provide human milk for their baby. Not being able to exclusively feed can be a big disappointment and a lot to have to adjust to, so mothers need encouragement and validation for their efforts in order to persevere.

Diabetes

Cases of type 1 diabetes have been rising, but the global incidence in children is very variable, from 0.1 cases per 100'000 in China, India and Venezuela to more than 60 cases per 100'000 in Finland (Atkinson et al, 2014). Most children are diagnosed with type 1 diabetes around the age of five to seven years, and there is another peak in presentation around the time of puberty. However, the number of diagnoses of diabetes are rising in the under two population, though very few are under six months.

Diabetes is a lifelong autoimmune disorder, and the goal of management is to keep blood glucose levels within a safe range, avoiding hypoglycaemia, which in young children, can lead to negative neurodevelopmental outcomes. The lactose in milk has been found to be around 70g per litre, which enables the mother and clinician to calculate the correct dose of insulin. One factor to bear in mind is that breastfed babies may have a different postprandial response to feeding, as human milk is higher in fat, which modulates the absorption of glucose, which may mean a less pronounced variability in blood sugar after a feed (Miller et al, 2017).

It may feel tempting for either a clinician or a mother to feed babies with expressed breast milk so that doses of insulin can be more accurately calculated. However, it is perfectly possible to encourage a mother to keep going with direct breastfeeding, using what we know about normal milk volumes – which is approximately 750ml in 24-hours.

If the infant feeds fairly regularly, then it may be possible to estimate the carbohydrate content by dividing the total 24-hour amount by the number of feeds. If, as with many babies, the feeds are more responsive and variable, then often the mother will instinctively know which feeds are larger (often the morning feed for example). Sometimes a very small feed would require such a small dose of insulin that it becomes impractical. Strategies such as test weighing can be utilised or measuring blood glucose levels regularly to ensure the child's blood sugar is maintained in their optimal range. Often, with some trial and error, a family can work out a routine that suits them best.

Of course, a multidisciplinary approach is particularly important with these children, to make sure that the family has access to all the right people, especially as solid foods are brought into the mix – working with the dietitian, paediatrician, clinical nurse specialist and lactation specialist, we can come up with creative solutions.

Sleepy babies

Many babies may struggle with somnolence, or sleepiness for many different reasons. Some of the most common reasons include being a late preterm or early term infant, infants with low tone, infants with higher metabolic rate or higher calorie needs who sleep more to conserve energy, as well as sick babies and those with jaundice.

Obviously, the underlying condition will need to be managed by the multidisciplinary team. If the infant is not exclusively receiving all their milk at the breast, the mother will also need to be supported to maintain their milk production. For those babies and children who are able to exclusively or partially receive some milk directly from the breast, certain feeding supports can help to optimise efficiency, maintain alertness and reduce stress to the infant.

It is especially important when babies are slow to get started with breastfeeding to offer plenty of skin-to-skin contact. Keeping a child skin to skin means that the child is in the right place to feed and there is no delay. It also maintains physiological stability and reduces stress – which will obviously support optimal feeding.

Many mothers, particularly mothers of babies with cardiac problems, find that upright feeding is really effective to help their infant stay awake during feeding (Lambert and Watters, 1998). Breast compressions can also be used to good effect to maximise milk intake and reduce effort for the child. Another good strategy is to encourage small, frequent feeds with rest breaks in between (Medoff-Cooper et al, 2010). If infants are stable and have enough tone, they may also be able to feed when lightly asleep. The only sleep state where feeding cannot occur is deep non-REM (slow wave) sleep when muscle tone is reduced, and feeding is physiologically impossible.

Post-operative children

Many parents are keen to comfort their babies and children after surgery, and technically, there is no reason why they cannot do this, provided that the post-operative instructions do not include continuing to be nil by mouth for clinical reasons. Once children have recovered from the effects of their anaesthetic, they are usually desperate to nurse, and once they show signs of readiness, they can feed. One strategy that is really supportive is to proactively inform mothers that they can breastfeed their child in recovery. Some mothers are unsure whether they are 'allowed' to do this, and being categorically told that this is encouraged is really supportive and validates this instinctive behaviour.

Many parents are concerned about hurting their child if they have a surgical incision or stitches, but they will probably have been given post-operative pain relief, so parents can be reassured about gently handling their children. Feeding also provides non-pharmacologic pain relief. I have lost count of the number of mothers who have told me that breastfeeding provided pain relief when all other painkillers failed to manage a child's discomfort.

Human milk is well-tolerated, and gastric emptying is rapid. Even so, antiemetics may be a pragmatic pre-emptive strategy to reduce the likelihood of vomiting. Most of the parents I support who have children with cancer (who have regular general anaesthetics not only for surgical intervention but also for procedures such as lumbar punctures [LPs]), report that if they wait until their child feels nauseous, it is far harder to get on top of the nausea with anti-emetics. Regular antiemetics seem to help children tolerate oral feedings better, but you will need to develop an individualised plan for feeding in collaboration with the paediatrician and dietitian if they are involved.

Sometimes, depending on the surgery, some creative positioning is required. Postoperatively, children may have drains, wounds, stomas, multiple lines, casts, or splints. Other times children need to be kept in a specific position. One mother I supported was nursing her 2-year-old who had a brain tumour, and following neurosurgery had to remain flat. This mother fed in a side-lying position or by dangle feeding, otherwise known as the wolf position, for several days while her daughter recovered.

218

Other times, due to the position of portacaths, Hickman lines, drains or surgical wounds, mothers end up feeding on one breast only. Sometimes they pump the other breast, and other times they are able to feed on the other side by rolling over so that they feed with the uppermost breast, squashing the other breast into the mattress. This clearly doesn't work for everyone, but for some mothers this has been found to ensure that both breasts are used and supply is maintained.

Another issue that crops up from time to time is that with large surgical wounds, sometimes a child is unable to be positioned in the way that is ideal. I have seen some pictures of breastfeeding positions that are far from 'textbook' but are adaptations to a large abdominal or chest wound which prevents a child from comfortably rolling onto their side. While not ideal, sometimes some tolerance for a less than perfect position is temporarily necessary.

Cleft lip/palate

Cleft lip and or palate can occur as part of a more global diagnosis, so these children may also have other problems with low tone, sleepiness or higher calorie intake. You may therefore need to use a combination of strategies. All children with cleft lip, cleft palate or cleft lip and palate will be seen by the cleft team, which will probably include some form of feeding support, though not always specialist lactation support.

Almost all mothers of children with clefts will need some lactation support. The problem with a cleft of the lip, and especially a cleft of the palate, is that infants will find it hard to create a vacuum. Milk may be dribbled out, not flow well, or may get into the cleft. Most will need to protect their supply initially by initiating early, effective exclusive pumping. Infants may need to be fed with a special needs feeder, or squeeze bottle.

Sometimes, an upright, forward position is helpful - using gravity as a positional aid. This is especially true if the infant also has sucking problems. Adopting a position where the mother leans back slightly, and has their infant positioned upright, straddling their lap means the baby will be upright and forward (Genna, 2017).

Babies with clefts usually need plenty of burp breaks due to excessive air intake. As infants transition to more oral feeds, thickening their milk may help them to swallow it, so involvement with the speech and language therapist is really essential. There is only patchy evidence that a palate prosthesis is helpful prior to surgical repair of a cleft, so more research is needed around that particular tool.

For infants with only a cleft of the lip, and where there are no other medical or neurological complications, if their mother has a very soft breast, it may be possible to manually occlude the cleft with the breast tissue to enable an effective seal.

A recent research study found that a cleft of the lip only was associated with greater rates of breastfeeding than clefts of the palate with or without a cleft of the lip. The type of cleft made no difference to the duration of providing milk with expressing (Madhoun et al, 2019), which is not a surprising finding if you think about it, provided that mothers have enough support and information on how to effectively maintain their supply with exclusive pumping.

Children with cancer

Infants and children with malignant disease can continue to breastfeed. The immunoglobulins present in human milk are especially beneficial for a child who is immunocompromised, providing protection against opportunistic viral and bacterial infections which could cause a child with cancer to develop an infection and febrile neutropaenia.

Human milk is not sterile, and it contains hundreds of strains of beneficial bacteria. Even for a neutropaenic child, there is no evidence that this is harmful. It does seem sensible to maintain additional hygiene precautions during profoundly neutropaenic episodes, washing hands before breastfeeding, and aiming to directly breastfeed when possible, rather than express and store milk.

Some children on treatment for cancer may require additional calories, or struggle to maintain weight due to loss of appetite, nausea and vomiting. Others may be too tired to feed effectively. They may therefore need either nasogastric tube feeding, supplemental feeds, or both. Some mothers may be able to borrow some of the techniques for increasing the calorie content of their milk that I mentioned earlier, such as giving extra fat rich milk, breast compressions and increasing their milk supply. Other children are prescribed fortifiers or high calorie formula to minimise excessive fluid intake. The details of how to manage the additional calories will need to be worked out between the family, paediatric oncologist, dietitian and lactation specialist.

There is no research regarding the theoretical risk of chemotherapy concentrations present in infant saliva being transferred to the mother via the backwash mechanism. This is known as the retrograde inoculation hypothesis with the infant's saliva seeding the human milk microbiome during breastfeeding (Beghetti et al, 2019). However, the amount of saliva is minimal, and the amount of chemotherapy present in the child's saliva is negligible. It would probably be prudent for a child on oral chemotherapy to take their chemotherapy after feeding, if possible, but IV chemotherapy would be unlikely to be passed via saliva to the maternal microbiome in problematic amounts.

In my informal survey and in the Breastfeeding the Brave support group that I am in contact with - at the time of writing - over 50 mothers are breastfeeding children from one month to five years who are receiving chemotherapy for various cancers. All continue to breastfeed, and no mothers have experienced any undue side effects. As an anecdotal tale, my own daughter had a fairly standard cocktail of chemotherapy, including intravenous, intramuscular, intrathecal and oral. I breastfed her with no restrictions throughout. Early in her treatment I became extremely fatigued and felt wiped out. I saw my own GP to rule out thyroid dysfunction and anaemia. But my energy levels improved significantly when I took greater care to use gloves after handling Filly's oral chemotherapy. I had been fairly blasé about her oral drugs, handling them with my bare hands and perhaps not always being careful to wash thoroughly. While breastfeeding her for 26 months did not affect my own health, handling her drugs without the due respect they deserved certainly did.

Clearly this is an area that needs further research, but at the present time, there does not appear to be any good reason to prevent a child from continuing to breastfeed, though this is an obvious research priority to provide more reassurance.

One area of caution is when a mother is caring for two children, or tandem nursing two – a baby and an older child. Depending on which child has cancer, there may be some creative workarounds such as assigning each child a breast to minimise saliva contamination, not feeding both children one after the other on the same breast or expressing milk for one of the children. These are not easy decisions. Care will also need to be taken when handling vomit and nappies from the child on chemotherapy. This is particularly important if both children are resident on the ward, as would be entirely appropriate if so desired by the family.

Breastfeeding may provide vital comfort and normality, it may be one of the only fluids or foods that are easily tolerated, and anecdotally, there appears to be much less incidence of painful mucositis (Thomas, 2020).

Sucking, swallowing, seal problems

I am indebted to Sarah Edney-Dutton and Stacey Zimmels for their expertise in this area. If oropharyngeal dysphagia is suspected, an urgent referral to a specialised SLT is essential, alongside lactation support. Some speech and language therapists are also dual qualified as IBCLCs and they have a wealth of knowledge in supporting children with sensorimotor or neurologically mediated feeding difficulties.

There are many sensorimotor problems that could affect the safety and efficacy of the suck-swallow-breathe sequence in infants and children. Some signs of oropharyngeal dysphagia include:

- Wet sounds or pooling secretions.
- Coughing, choking, or gagging.
- Breast refusal or irritability.
- Unusually long or short feeds.
- Faltering growth.
- Colour changes or apnoeas.
- Increased work of breathing.
- Posturing e.g., arching or neck extension.

Obviously, there is a balance with these children to maintain the safety of their swallow and airway, alongside the risks and benefits of continuing to breastfeed. Depending on the severity of the condition, it may be possible to continue to breastfeed with support and monitoring, or for some children suckling a well-drained breast while being nasogastric tube fed may be clinically appropriate (Kruger et al, 2019; Lawlor & Choi, 2020; Ongkasuwan & Chiou, 2018).

One of the most often utilised tests to assess the safety of the swallow is a video fluoroscopy which uses X-ray while a child swallows. You may remember Emma's story in Chapter 4 of the child with the severe airway condition. The downside of this test, as Emma found, was that it is not useful to assess breastfeeding, as the child cannot be actively breastfeeding during the procedure. A more appropriate test is fibreoptic endoscopic evaluation of swallowing (FEES) in which a child may continue to breastfeed, and the full feed can be imaged (Willette et al, 2016). Unfortunately, FEES is not available in every unit, so this is not an approach that will be an option for all families.

Critically sick children

I'm grateful to Dr Vicky Thomas for many discussions over the years with respect to supporting very sick breastfed children. While it may seem obvious to many clinicians, we do need to consider the impact of feeding and milk on the sickest children. When children require intensive care, they are usually critically ill or unstable. Most of these children will be fully ventilated, and therefore they are unable to breastfeed. Indeed, some children who are critically unwell are neither orally nor enterally fed. While nutrition is important, and children need to continue to grow, when they are profoundly unwell, this is not the priority.

It is extremely important that while feeding is not a clinical priority to the child who is unconscious, unstable or critically unwell, it continues to be a family centred care priority. In other words, just because the child cannot breastfeed, or even tolerate a full nasogastric feed, the mother should be encouraged to continue to express milk, valuing the importance of this milk, and reminding the mother that when the child recovers, they will be able to breastfeed again.

When a child is this unstable or unwell, although they usually do not receive full feeds, their hydration and fluid balance, as well as their electrolyte balance is extremely important. They are usually kept on clear IV fluids to maintain their hydration and blood sugar levels, as well as certain electrolytes such as potassium. They may also receive trophic feeds, which are intended to keep the gut moving and healthy, rather than to facilitate growth and weight gain. These trophic feeds are of very low volume and expressed breast milk may be used. Occasionally, children receive Total Parenteral Nutrition (TPN), but this depends on their condition, and a recent trial (PEPaNIC) found that there is an increased risk of infection and poorer neurodevelopmental outcomes when TPN is used in the first week of acute illness (Verstraete et al, 2019).

One intervention that can be recommended is to use expressed breast milk for mouth care, and ideally, parents could get involved with this. This can be a good way to validate the importance and meaning of breast milk at a time when a mother may be distressed that she cannot directly breastfeed. Sick children also benefit from loving touch and holding if clinically stable and able to tolerate this.

Of course, the parents of critically sick children are very likely to be upset, stressed, and anxious about their child. Their condition may be known and expected, or it could be sudden – such as a traumatic accident, sudden onset of illness or injury/burn. A huge amount of compassion and sensitive communication is needed. Mothers usually realise that their child cannot breastfeed when they are very unwell, but they may need support to continue to express, and overcome the impacts of stress and trauma on their milk ejection reflex. They may also need support to store their milk, protect their milk supply, and facilitate the return to direct breastfeeding once their child begins to recover.

As a child recovers, they can slowly work up to receiving larger amounts of feed. It may be sensible to use the freshest breast milk possible, to maximise the immunologic benefits to the child. Ideally, the paediatrician, nursing team, dietitian, speech and language therapist, and mother should work collaboratively to return the child back to breastfeeding. Any feeding plans should also be communicated clearly to staff in other wards if the child is transferred to the High Dependency Unit or stepped down to the general children's ward. You may wish to go back to the section on returning to oral feeding after extubation and enteral feeding, as well as read about the impacts of iatrogenic withdrawal as well.

One major gap in the research that I have mentioned a few times is skin-to-skin care of critically ill children in the PICU. There is an abundance of literature relating to this being a supportive intervention in preterm neonates. There is no sensible reason why skin-to-skin for fully ventilated preterm babies can be facilitated and yet is seen as impossible for older babies. This is mostly a matter of culture that can and should be challenged. Of course, as is the case with some very unwell and unstable neonates, skin to skin is not appropriate for every child, all of the time. However, we really should be shifting our thinking towards seeing this as standard care. I have heard many parents describe how distressed and disempowered they feel when they are not able to touch, hold and comfort their very sick children. At a time when breastfeeding is (necessarily) not feasible, we should prioritise touch and closeness as far as clinically appropriate and practical. I appreciate that some children have a history of dislodging their endotracheal or tracheostomy tube, or are too unstable to move. However, if we start from the position of 'why *shouldn't* this child be held', or 'when *can* this child be held', we will begin to slowly shift towards an expectation of close contact as the norm, and an absence of touch as a deviation from standard care.

Test yourself:

1. For babies with low tone, which of the following strategies is NOT usually recommended?

   a. Dancer hand position.

   b. Upright feeding.

   c. Judicious use of a nipple shield.

   d. A 4-hourly feeding routine.

2. Which babies are LEAST likely to become fatigued during feeding at the breast?

   a. Babies with Down syndrome.

   b. Babies with cardiac defects.

   c. Babies with cleft palate.

   d. Babies with phenylketonuria.

3. Which strategies may support more efficient feeding?

   a. Breast compressions.

   b. Frequent feeding.

   c. Upright feeding.

   d. All the above.

4. When children are too sick to breastfeed, which is the *most* important aspect of care apart from ensuring the infant is adequately nourished?

   a. Protect the maternal milk supply.

   b. Reassure the mother that they have done a great job.

   c. Suggest the mother catch up on sleep.

   d. Provide the mother with handouts on how to reduce milk supply.

Chapter 10

Emotional, practical and family centred support

Family centred care (FCC) is a term that is neither well defined, nor implemented in practice. For a start, there is no absolute definition of what FCC is, although there are some agreed principles:

- Information sharing.
- Respecting and honouring differences.
- Partnerships and collaboration.
- Negotiation.
- Care in the context of the family and community.

The most recent Cochrane review (Shields et al, 2012) found that there is very little high-quality evidence about how FCC can be implemented and what the benefits are.

Family centred care is relatively new, and perhaps this is why it is slow to get off the ground. We must remember that it used to be common practice until as late as the 1980's for children to be resident in hospitals without their parents. William Goldfarb extensively researched the impact of separation of children and parents mostly from a foster care perspective (Goldfarb, 1943). It was Rene Spitz and Katherine Wolf who first began to challenge the practice of separating children and parents (Spitz, 1945; Spitz and Wolf, 1946). They produced a film called 'Grief: A Peril in Infancy' documenting the effects of separating mothers and children in the first year of life. (You can still watch this on YouTube - though it is distressing viewing.) There were multiple researchers at the time exploring attachment and bonding, including Harry Harlow (1949; 1958) Harlow and Zimmermann (1959), Bowlby et al (1952) and Bowlby (1960). On the back of all this research, came the Platt Report, which essentially argued that parents and children should not be separated in hospitals (Platt, 1959; 1962).

However, the Platt report recommendations were not fully implemented into practice until as late as the 1980's, with adolescent services being particularly late to adopt the principles of FCC. In 1982, less than half of all children's wards had open access for parents, and many children were still being cared for on adult wards.

When we consider that many hospital buildings predate the full implementation of the Platt report, it is perhaps easier to understand why the infrastructure itself does not lend itself to FCC. Long 'Nightingale' style wards and small isolation cubicles are not ideal for allowing families to remain together. Many of these Nightingale wards have been refurbished, and yet what seems to have happened in many cases is that they were carved up into small cubicles that are not set up as a family-sized space. Yet, with some creativity and open mindedness, many hospitals have managed to be flexible, although this is far from standardised. I have spoken to parents up and down the country and some report exemplary FCC, while others are seriously suboptimal.

FCC is at the heart of paediatric healthcare delivery, including the critical care environment (Young et al, 2006), but both in practice and according to the literature, this is sometimes hard to achieve, particularly when it comes to collaborative decision-making, person-centred communication and treating parents with empathy (Terp et al, 2021). FCC involves positioning the parents as experts in their child's care, collaborating with the family as partners, and sharing information (see figure 1 below).

Figure 1: What does FCC look like in the paediatric environment?

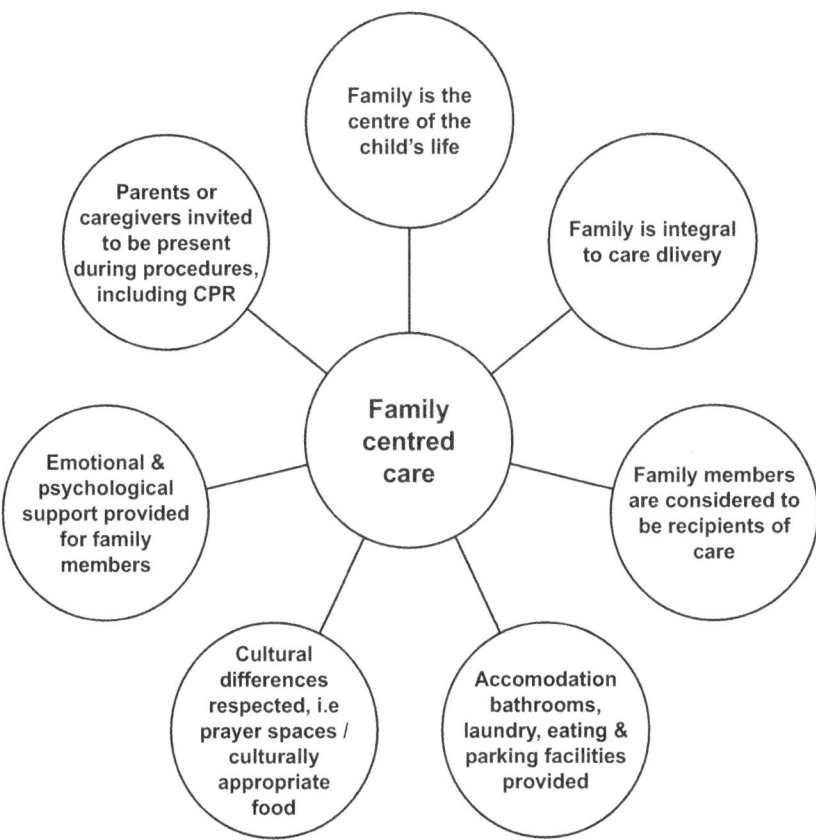

Some studies have found that parents do not feel as involved as they would have liked when their child is in a critical care environment (Ames et al, 2011; Butler et al, 2014; Hill et al, 2019; Terp et al, 2021). There are also additional pressures relating to parenting in a very public environment – especially when a child is in intensive care, where the clinical environment is usually very open (Rempel et al, 2013).

How is FCC relevant to breastfeeding?

You may already realise how interrelated FCC and breastfeeding are. In case it is not obvious, I find it helpful to remember that we need to meet *all* of people's needs in order for them to thrive. When it comes to the often 'sacrificial' act of breastfeeding, mothers need to be relieved of stress and have their presence valued in order for them to successfully breastfeed.

So how do we meet these needs and reduce stress for parents? There may be many answers to this, but here are my suggestions:

- Valuing parent's expertise (you might be the expert on their condition, but they are the experts on how their child responds to that condition).
- Positioning parents as part of the team.
- Provide choices.
- Acts of kindness.
- Welcome.
- Maintain dignity.
- Preserve normality.
- Understand the stressors:
- Other children.
- Finances.
- Accommodation.
- Food and drink.
- Liaising with employers.
- Protecting sleep.
- Facilitating bedsharing.

I will delve into the practicalities of these principles throughout this chapter. They are all important in order to reduce the chance of the parent feeling redundant, not being fully informed, and the trauma (including vicarious trauma) of observing illness, as well as the psychological and practical challenges of parenting in a 'goldfish bowl' environment.

What families need

Supporters of the family of a sick child are often blindsided by news of the illness, and forget that often families need practical care, emotional support and some normality. While it's easy for non-medics to feel powerless, often what families need is not more medical information, but love and support. Having a wide array of tools and ideas with which to support families can make a big difference to their hospital experience.

Clinicians in hospitals can sometimes become immune to the horror of critical illness – often this is an understandable coping mechanism. When we see sick children every day, it is easy to forget that for a family, this may be the most worrying or distressing experience they have ever had. Lactation professionals and those with counselling backgrounds may find the emotional aspects of caring for a family more intuitive, and yet may still need a prompt to understand which suggestions may be supportive.

This chapter focuses on the non-clinical aspects of care of families. Within it you will find information about how to meet the practical, emotional and psychological needs of families caring for a medically complex child in hospital.

How to support a sick child and their family in hospital

First and foremost, for most families, the hospital is a scary place. It's easy to become desensitised to the environment that we work in every day as clinicians. I think we have done a tremendous amount to try to support children through the fear of hospitals, but perhaps we sometimes forget that it's scary for parents too. Therefore, for the sake of both parents and children, try to safeguard normality as much as possible.

Encourage families to keep as many of their usual routines as they can, provide emotional support, or refer parents for this if you are too busy. Also, try to keep families together as much as possible, including during procedures. I have spoken to many parents who were not allowed to be with their children during painful procedures, and this can be very worrying for both parent and child. It is likely that parents will want to be with their children during procedures, and breastfeeding is a comfort measure that can provide reassurance as well as nurture and pain relief for children.

I think it's worth remembering that there is never a good time for illness to strike, so bear in mind that parents may be worried and preoccupied with the many tasks they probably left undone, the other children they have at home, their work, partner, pets, and many other normal day-to-day tasks and activities that need to go on hold when a child is admitted to hospital. Life cannot simply go on hold – so for most parents, a hospital admission means dropping all the balls they were juggling and making hasty and thrown-together plans. While none of those stresses are technically the responsibility of the clinicians caring for children, bear in mind that parents are often stressed not just because of the obvious reason, but the unseen and less obvious ones as well. While resident on the paediatric ward, parents may not be able to access their usual stress management coping strategies either - such as exercise, walking the dog, taking their weekly swim or Pilates class, or whatever else is their go-to stressbuster. This means that their mental health may be taking a hit, not only because of the acute stress of the situation but also because they are unable to manage their mental health in their preferred way.

Most people would agree that play therapy and play provision for children in hospital is fantastic and continues to be a wonderful tool to distract, aid understanding of procedures, demystify treatment, and provide a welcome opportunity to pursue the normal activities of childhood. After all, play is the work of childhood and so, whenever developmentally and clinically appropriate, encourage play for your little patients. It's also a way for parents to behave normally and it can feel grounding and reassuring for them to see their child playing.

I have thought for some time that we almost need the equivalent of 'play therapy' for adults too (don't worry, I'm not talking about blowing bubbles or organised games here). If you can, try to remind parents to do activities that make *them* feel better. For some this may be something they can do with their hands – such as doodling, drawing, colouring, knitting, or fiddling with fidget toys. For others they may need to distract their minds – perhaps doing a crossword, sudoku, playing solitaire on their phone, or working on a puzzle book. Other parents prefer reading, listening to music or an audiobook or watching a movie. Self-care is important therapy for parents. If they are running on empty, they are less able to be emotionally available for their child. So, in caring for parents, you are caring for your patients.

It's also a good idea to maintain calm, and minimise interventions overnight, which I will return to in a moment.

Involving parents

The involvement of parents in their children's care can be a hard balance to get right. This should not be interpreted as 'delegating tasks' to parents to reduce nursing workload. I have spoken to parents who have ended up doing their child's clinical observations or managing all their NG feeds. Certainly, parents can be empowered to be involved with some clinical tasks (Flacking et al, 2007), but firstly, the clinical oversight should always be with a clinician – it is an unfair level of responsibility for a parent to feel that it is their job to monitor their child. Secondly, the parent's primary role is to be a parent, not to 'switch sides' and become their child's nurse. There is perhaps no easy answer to balancing this, but here are some suggestions:

- Ask parents how they wish to be involved.
- Provide choices and flexibility.
- Always assume that clinical tasks are a clinician's responsibility, and allocate time for this. Never use a parent for unofficial nursing tasks – consider them supernumerary if this helps with time management. This will also ensure patient safety.
- Do not assume that just because parents are competent, that they always wish to have the task fall to them. I have heard parents whose child is long term tube fed express a wish for respite from this task while in hospital. Just because they do a task all the time does not mean they always want to do it.
- Anecdotally, many parents who are also healthcare professionals sometimes fall into the familiar role of medical or nursing care. While this is sometimes a stress-response, keep in mind that this may not be the best way to handle the situation, and encourage them to take ownership of the more 'normal' aspects of caring for their child.
- Keep the negotiation fluid – how a parent wishes to be involved in their child's care today may not be the same as yesterday, or tomorrow.

- Ask them how much information they need. Many clinicians are natural teachers, but parents do not always have the capacity for lengthy or technical explanations. Equally, some parents feel more in control if they are provided with more information.

Painful procedures

When children have painful or invasive procedures, it is important to offer parents choices, if possible, about whether they can be present. Many parents describe not being able to be with their child during blood tests, cannulation, nasopharyngeal aspirates, LPs and other procedures, as traumatic. If parents are separated from their children, they are often stressed or deeply anxious when they hear their child cry out and are unable to comfort them.

Sometimes parents are told they cannot be present because they will find it too upsetting, but the reality is that hearing their child in distress is equally, if not more, upsetting for many parents. We should not make assumptions about what a parent wants to do.

Another plausible reason is that some healthcare professionals are put off by having parents present. This is even more the case if the clinician is being taught or supervised by a senior colleague. While I understand this from a human perspective, nothing justifies separating a parent and child during a distressing procedure if it will offer even a small amount of comfort or reassurance to either the child, parent or both. My pragmatic suggestion is to ensure parents know where to stand, and give them a space to be with their child where they can offer reassurance without accidentally knocking over the LP sample bottles or whatever.

Ultimately, some parents may choose to stay out of the room, but it is always better to offer a choice. I still regret not pushing to be allowed to be present for my eldest child's LP when she was admitted with meningitis at ten months. The sound of her crying from the procedure room down the corridor haunted me for many months. It is far better for many parents to know they offered all the comfort they could, rather than to worry that they might have been able to reduce their child's suffering in even a small way by being present.

Finally, breastfeeding can offer some pain relief and many mothers report feeling upset or dismissed when their offer to breastfeed their child during a blood test or cannula insertion is refused. While the current evidence has only explored breastfeeding as pain relief for immunisation and heel sticks (Shah et al., 2015; Harrison et al., 2016), anecdotally many mothers find that it offers effective pain relief for other procedures as well. I would suggest listening open mindedly to mothers and giving them options about how they can offer breastfeeding as a comfort measure. In some scenarios it is logistically difficult or impossible to breastfeed at the same time – such as during nasogastric tube insertion or a throat swab. Other times it may affect safety or precision, such as during an LP. At those times, breastfeeding can be offered immediately post-procedure for comfort if the mother is physically present, and comfort during the procedure can be provided to the child in other ways – such as stroking, hand-holding, play therapy or distraction, singing or reading a story.

One word of caution is that some mothers are fiercely protective of breastfeeding as a positive parenting tool and do not wish it to be commandeered by healthcare staff as a way to facilitate easier cannulation or blood tests. A few mothers have told me that they resented clinicians asking them if they would breastfeed in order to make cannulation easier. The subtle difference here is perhaps that those clinicians were asking the mother to breastfeed because it made *their* job easier, rather than primarily thinking about what was best for the mother and child. As is so often the case, the key is to ask mothers for their preference and provide choices.

Emotional and practical support

To provide emotional and practical support, encouragement is an obvious recommendation, but co-creation of feeding plans with families will help them feel involved and their expertise about their child acknowledged. Families have innate wisdom, and know their child's likes and dislikes. They also have instinct. When health professionals defer to parents' instinct it sends a strong message of empowerment that they too can trust that instinct. After all, instinct may have been what helped them to realise there was a problem with their child in the first place.

It's also important to value human milk and consider it as both part of the medicine to make their child well, and also part of the normality that links them with home life. When health professionals demonstrate with words and actions that breast milk is important, it helps mothers feel motivated to continue.

Finally, there may be practical stressors, such as finances or work. When families are stressed by these practical matters it may primarily affect their ability and energy levels to care for their child at a difficult time, but it also may be a barrier to continuing to provide breast milk. Clearly the NHS doesn't have a limitless budget for charitable giving, but there may be referrals for additional support, access to charity funds, hospital accommodation, parking ticket exemptions, and letters of support to employers that can be offered to assist families.

Sometimes a social worker, health visitor or a volunteer can be referred to for support with filling in forms like application for disability allowance and so on. It's a depressing form to fill out, as the child's worst days have to be considered, and I found during my years as a health visitor that many parents are naturally optimistic, and then sometimes get their disability allowance application rejected. Support to fill out this lengthy and complex document is highly valued by families.

Other children

Another major area of stress for many families is the worry they may have over other children at home. It can feel like a real wrench to be away from other children, especially if this is a relatively long admission. It's also worth considering whether other children at home are also being breastfed. It may be highly stressful for families with other children, whether they are breastfed or not, and many mothers feel very torn, between wanting to be with their unwell child, but also feeling like they have abandoned their other child or children. This can cause a high level of stress and upset, and while there is not always anything that health professionals can do, we can always ask about other children, and show that we care how families are managing.

For more chronic conditions, psychological support is often available for siblings – for example music or art therapy, or the sibling may be able to access some talking therapy or play therapy. Siblings can be a huge source of comfort, normality and support to each other, they are often caring, fun and an always available playmate. For these and many other reasons, at some times, it may be appropriate to consider whether there is a way to keep families together.

Keeping families together

It is not always possible or appropriate, and I'm not suggesting that for a short admission this would always be practical, but there is an argument for considering how families can be kept together. This is particularly relevant for longer term admissions where one parent is working, there is no local family to care for another sibling, or both children are being breastfed, like one mother I met who was tandem nursing her 8-month-old baby alongside his three-year-old sister with a Stage 4 Wilms tumour.

There may be creative solutions, such as finding a larger room or cubicle, pushing two beds together, and facilitating bedsharing. Allowing siblings to stay needn't be the huge barrier that we might think it is. Even allowing partners to stay, particularly if the situation is very distressing, a child is critically unwell, or the primary caregiver is exhausted.

I appreciate that all units are different and may have different logistical or practical constraints but facilitating FCC has been achieved in other areas, such as neonatal intensive care, and perhaps it's time within paediatrics to adopt a creative, curious and can-do approach, rather than defaulting to the position that partners and siblings may not stay overnight.

Allowing partners to stay may be particularly important when a child is extremely unwell, their condition is evolving or deteriorating, or the primary carer is exhausted or unwell themselves. Allowing another family member to remain may be difficult due to space constraints, but it may be a compassionate response in specific circumstances.

My name is not Mum or Dad

Another area I, and many others feel strongly about is referring to parents by their names, rather than the generic 'mum' or 'dad' which is so common (Nimmo, 2019). Firstly, many parents feel invisible when they are referred to by the relationship they have to your patient. Outside of this situation, they have many other roles, responsibilities, skills and identities. The only people who earn the right to call parents 'Mum' or 'Dad' are the children of those people. For many parents, this generic use of the same name can feel patronising and 'othering'. Instead, ask parents what they wish to be called.

Secondly, not all parents identify with the name Mum or Dad, particularly transgender or non-binary identifying parents. Others may have a difficult relationship with their own mother or father and find these words triggering. Same sex parents may have different words for themselves and using the word 'Mum' or 'Dad' may cause confusion when there are other adult visitors around whose relationship to the child is not immediately obvious. I have cared for many same sex parents who got utterly despondent when staff assumed they were a friend, sister or aunty, rather than the other mum. This is also true for step-parents or partners of the primary carer who do not wish to be called 'Mum' or 'Dad'.

I know it's hard to remember names, and many health care professionals defer to the name Mum or Dad because they can't hold lots of names in their head – after all, it can be hard enough to remember your patients' names. So, a few ways that you might make this easier for yourself include:

- Providing name badges for parents (make sure these are large enough for long names).
- Writing their names on a whiteboard above the child's bed space.
- Including their name in handover.
- Writing the parents name on the front of the medical file and observation charts so it's readily available.

If you worry that you will forget, I assure you that most parents are utterly forgiving if you need to ask them to remind you. They would mostly far rather you apologised for forgetting their name and asked for a reminder, than defaulted back to Mum or Dad. This also applies if you have trouble pronouncing a name that is unfamiliar. Please just ask. This small extra effort goes a long way to individualising care and helping parents feel 'seen' and valued.

Caring for parents is part of good paediatric care

When I surveyed health care professionals, almost all of them felt that supporting parents to achieve their breastfeeding goals was an important part of their job. Of course, supporting a parent with their feeding goals is just one part of supporting parents in general, but it is important to remember that breastfeeding is incredibly important to families, and also as a public health intervention.

Broadly speaking, caring for parents means that they will be in a better position to care for their children, so ask how they are coping and remember that even short admissions are traumatising and disruptive for some people. Encourage parents to swap out with trusted friends, family members or partners to get breaks if they can organise this, and praise and encourage them. It's hard to parent in a public place, and just *existing* on a paediatric ward is very difficult, especially when it is for more than a few days. Parents are often stoical, but they may be fiercely trying to hold it all together underneath the outward display of resilience.

Also, remember practicality. Ask if parents have enough food, or the means to obtain or cook food. This includes ensuring that parents with allergies, intolerances, or cultural/religious food preferences are provided with practical food options. It is not enough to provide a vegan mother with a portion of chips and a salad for example. On a related note, snacks should also be available. Think about how often we go to the fridge or cupboard if we are home? We do not simply eat three meals a day. Plentiful snacks and drinks should be provided for families so they are not forced to supplement a meagre food offering with whatever they can find in the vending machine or overpriced on-site hospital shop.

I'm sure paediatric professionals know about Ronald MacDonald and other hospital accommodation options for parents whose children are admitted to a tertiary specialist centre far from home, but lactation professionals may not be aware that finding accommodation close to the hospital may be possible to enable families to stay together. These houses provide on-site accommodation to families whose children have been hospitalised and also provide parents with a palace to cook and eat, as well as get away from the stressful hospital environment.

Finally, make time to talk to parents as fellow adults. It is exceptionally lonely to be a parent of a sick child for days, weeks or months on end. It is also quite amazing how much of oneself is lost while resident with a child in a paediatric ward. The professionals who make time to care about how a parent is coping, make a joke, or make small talk honestly are up there in some professional hall of fame in a parent's eyes.

Practical breast care for lactating mothers

One really obvious way that we need to care for mothers better is when they have a breast-related problem while their child is resident on the paediatric ward. Mothers may have a breast condition that is directly related to their child's condition, or it may be unrelated. Either way, it can be difficult for mothers to access timely support and breast care while they are caring for their sick child.

It is common for mothers whose child is not feeding well to develop engorgement, blocked ducts and mastitis as a direct result of their child not draining the breast as well as usual. An obvious need for many mothers is to be given a breast pump to use. These need to be designated to the paediatric ward as well as the ED so that nobody has to borrow them from the postnatal or neonatal wards, and mothers do not need to wait. There also needs to be more than one breast pump. I have had many mothers tell me that the breast pump they were using was taken away for another mother or prioritised for a younger baby. There needs to be an adequate number of pumps. We wouldn't dream of not having enough oxygen saturation monitors or drip stands in the equipment cupboard. So why is it different for breast pumps?

Some mothers may also need urgent medical care to treat mastitis, abscess, or worrying breast lumps. Please consider asking medical colleagues who deal with adults to come to the paediatric ward or PICU to see mothers as 'outliers' rather than expect them to go to the emergency department and wait to be seen. It is hugely stressful for mothers to be separated from their children. There are also many clinical protocols that can guide clinical decision making, such as those on engorgement and mastitis (Mitchell et al, 2022), breast pain (Berens et al, 2016), breast lumps (Mitchell et al, 2019) and hyperlactation (Johnson et al, 2020).

Another common scenario is the parent (whether lactating or not) who needs emergency medication. I remember vividly that soon after my youngest child was diagnosed with cancer, the sinusitis that I had been ignoring for several days became excruciating. I won't bore you with gory details but suffice it to say I needed antibiotics and some more sensible pain relief. The specialist cancer hospital was an hour's drive across London from my GP, and I couldn't have left my three-year-old at such a difficult time for her anyway. Thankfully my GP agreed to assess me over the phone and leave a prescription at our local pharmacy for my husband to collect and bring to me the next day. But how would this have worked if I were a single parent, or my partner did not drive or have the means to get across town? What if a parent didn't realise that this was an option and sat and suffered in silence? It made me wonder – how could we make these scenarios easier for parents? Whether they need an anti-inflammatory for back pain, paracetamol for fever, or have run out of their antidepressants, we should be able to get them access to medical care without unnecessary delay. This is especially important for parents whose children are long term patients, for single parents who have limited options when it comes to swapping with someone else, those with disabilities, no transport, or in a hospital far from home because leaving the ward is really not an easy or viable option.

Impact on parents and families of having a sick child

Although there is a lack of research relating to the specific impacts of illness on breastfeeding, there is plentiful research relating to the impact of child illness and hospitalisation on families in general. One qualitative study found that both children and parents reported shock, sadness, confusion, frustration, and anger. Parents additionally experience feelings of numbness and worry (Gannoni and Shute, 2010).

Stress, trauma and anxiety are also frequently described by parents (Mortensen et al, 2015; Muscara et al, 2015; Foster et al, 2017) and other research recommends that parents are provided with adequate psychological support during hospitalisation of their child for a life-threatening condition (Smith et al, 2015; Pelentsov et al, 2015). Some parents develop post-traumatic stress disorder after watching their child becoming profoundly unwell, witnessing their child's resuscitation, or receiving a diagnosis of a life-threatening disease or condition (Woolf et al, 2016) and this has similarly been found in the neonatal intensive care unit as well (Malouf et al, 2022). Make sure that parents are aware that they can access support to help them process these difficult feelings and let them know how to arrange this after their child is home again, as some parents describe these feelings being most burdensome after discharge from hospital.

Some evidence suggests that chronic conditions lasting more than three months, and requiring multiple hospitalisations or medical treatments are more stressful for families. However, interestingly, the severity of a child's illness does not always seem to be a factor in predicting parental stress (Franck et al, 2010).

Childhood illness can be very disruptive to family life. Indeed, some research has found that it is the disruption to normal activities of daily living that causes the most distress, rather than the uncertainty of diagnosis. One study exploring the stressors experienced by children with a cancer diagnosis and their parents found that both children and parents found the disruption to normal life more stressful than the diagnosis itself (Rodriguez et al, 2012). This study also found that parental stress was significantly higher if they had children aged five and younger - mainly due to the uncontrollability of some of the aspects of caregiving. From personal experience I suspect this is also because they usually are less self-sufficient and require more intense parenting, play and distraction. Providing care to a child who is chronically unwell presents many psychological difficulties, but it can also have a profound effect on parenting confidence and self-efficacy, as well as limit setting and discipline (Mitchell et al, 2020). Parents may value the chance to discuss the challenges of limit setting and discussing their frustration over their child's behaviour without feeling like everyone is watching and judging. Whether children are sick or not, sometimes they have challenging behaviour, and this can feel particularly hard to handle in the confines of the paediatric ward.

Let parents know that good parenting does not always mean perfectly even-tempered, and that everyone reaches their limit sometimes.

There are also many practical and logistical problems associated with having a sick child, such as needing to have time off work, adaptations to lifestyle, relationship strain and loneliness and isolation for the parent resident with the hospitalised child. While the resident parent and child are on the ward, they are unable to access usual sources of companionship, activities, entertainment and exercise, and it is often harder or impractical for other siblings to visit – causing parents to make difficult choices about which child they have most contact with (Ivany et al, 2016; Belanger et al, 2017). Some research has also found that the parents of chronically unwell and disabled children are also themselves more likely to experience poor health (Vonneilich et al, 2016) possibly due to chronic stress, and exacerbated by delaying seeking personal support and care due to prioritising caring for their child.

It is common for parents to struggle with finances and income, and this affects those with lower incomes disproportionately (Beck et al, 2017). While admitted to a ward or unit, parents often have to purchase food for themselves or their child, and the on-site hospital shopping facilities are often more expensive (Thomson et al, 2016). Some parents may need to give up paid employment to care for their child (Kish et al, 2018), while others have to make adaptations or rely on understanding employers – which adds to their stress. On top of this, parents may have to pay for transport, parking, travel for other family members and associated costs of being away from home. It is hard to maintain usual duties such as laundry, housework and caring for other children while resident on the ward. Juggling work, wider family members, a partner, the home and pets is difficult and stressful, and has an indirect effect on parental mental health and coping ability (van Oers et al, 2014).

Practical tips and hacks

Bearing in mind what we know about how stressful it is to have a sick child, there are many practical ways that you can reduce the stress and mental load for parents. This may be particularly important for those whose children have chronic illness or disability and may attend hospital frequently. A list of suggestions, or a leaflet with some tips to help parents navigate hospital admission may be really welcome. Naturally parents figure these hacks out eventually for themselves, but it really takes the stress out if you can pre-empt some of the common challenges.

Firstly, it's a good idea for a mother to bring a manual pump with them if they have one. It's not a perfect substitute for a decent double electric hospital grade pump, but in an emergency, if a pump wasn't available, it would be very welcome. Many mothers keep theirs in a Tupperware container and leave it in their bag.

Another hack I personally found particularly useful when navigating frequent admissions with very little warning is to set up a WhatsApp group for sibling care which works like a cascade. One text or call to the group initiates everyone else in the group negotiating among themselves who is available to collect and care for a sibling, or a pet for that matter, which means that this is one less thing to be anxious about.

It's also helpful to have a designated person who can communicate specific needs or difficulties to people and take the organisational load off the parent's plate. This may also include interventions like a meal train. Although some breastfeeding mothers are provided with food on the paediatric ward, firstly this is inconsistent across units, and secondly, sometimes they would rather have a home cooked meal. There is something that feels incredibly nurturing about being brought a meal. It involves the community and although many parents are keen to show they can cope and get on with things, asking for and accepting help is not a sign of weakness, and also provides a valuable opportunity for members of the wider family and community to help and get involved.

Another tip is that some adult life insurance with critical illness cover will pay a significant lump sum if a child is diagnosed with certain life-threatening conditions. While it can feel rather vulgar to think about money at a time of trauma, unfortunately, money becomes a very real and practical problem and source of stress for families of children with chronic or significant illnesses and in some cases, the lump sum is enough to reduce the stress of needing to take unpaid leave or take some time off work to care for a sick child.

One tip that is borrowed from my time working as the FCC coordinator in a large NICU is to take a leaf out of hotel reception books, and keep a supply of essentials somewhere, ready to provide for families who have left home in a hurry. Sometimes children deteriorate quickly, and parents forget essential items. Having a supply of toothbrushes, toothpaste, combs, deodorant, sanitary supplies, breast pads and universal phone chargers is a really practical and thoughtful idea that makes a big difference to stressed families.

Finally, many families whose children have long term health problems keep a pre-packed hospital bag in the car, or by the front door in case of an emergency dash to hospital. For some families, the distance to hospital is significant, so popping home to grab another shirt or the phone charger is just not practical. If frequent hospitalisation is expected, this takes one task out of the equation.

Hospital bag

It may be really helpful to have a list of recommended items to pack in a hospital bag. Many families in a crisis have a bit of a brainstorm and can't remember what things they will need to bring. It's not patronising to ensure that families have the items that will be essential for them. One tip is to pack the main bag, but then also have a couple of grab bags with changes of clothes for child and parent so that the parent visiting from home can bring the grab bag and swap it out for dirties when they visit, then launder the clothes and repack the capsule bag. It can be very difficult to manage dirty laundry on the ward. Not all wards and units have laundry facilities, and with some wards being boiling hot and others being freezing cold, not to mention caring for children with vomiting and nausea - it can be hard to stay comfortable and fresh.

Another good tip is to pack ear plugs – hospitals are exceptionally noisy places. Phone chargers, kindles and iPads are also useful for staying connected and entertained. Depending on the age of the child, some favourite games might be lifesavers, and for younger children, bringing small activities to while away long and boring hours on the ward are invaluable.

It's also a good idea to pack non-perishable snacks – popcorn, dried fruit and nuts, granola bars and sachets of hot chocolate or herbal tea bags to enable the resident parent to have their favourite hot drink, rather than hospital issue coffee! Caution parents about valuables such as iPads, tablets, kindles, laptops and smartphones. It's really sad that this happens, but personal items can and do get stolen from paediatric wards. I remember many years ago, before the Patientline TVs were installed as standard, that the children's isolation cubicles used to have a physical TV. I was always stunned at how many of these were stolen. If people can walk out of the hospital with a TV, a laptop is no problem at all.

Remember contact lens solution, breast pads and sanitary products as well – it's inconvenient to be caught without these, and also suggest that parents have an emergency supply of painkillers that are in a child safe bottle. There's nothing worse than having a splitting headache on the paediatric ward – it's really not that easy to get hold of a couple of ibuprofen if you're not the actual patient. Parents may also wish to have certain items that are essential for sleep, such as an extra pillow, lavender spray or an eye mask. If nothing else, lavender makes a welcome change from the general hospital smells! As bizarre as this sounds, I always used to pack my favourite Neals Yard moisturiser, as I found the scent deeply soothing to my jangled nerves.

Remind parents not to forget things like a notebook to write down questions, and a comfort object for their child if they are attached to a particular toy.

But finally, everyone is human, and things do get forgotten. Having some essentials available means that parents are not caught on the back foot or stressed without something they really need.

Communicating with families

When communicating with families, while we don't want to overthink the complexities of their lives, it's worth remembering that we don't know half of what many people are dealing with behind the scenes. There may be many things that parents can't or don't want to tell us. They are also probably exhausted and even if they happen to be well informed or health professional parents, this is a stressful situation, so provide simple explanations and detail, and in a variety of different forms so parents can revisit the information later.

Some ideas for this include writing things down, drawing pictures, or encouraging the parent to record a voice note so they can replay it later, or with a partner. It can be hard for parents to recall conversations for partners that are not present during the ward round, so check understanding, or offer to come back later if it is a difficult diagnosis. Single parents may need more emotional support from staff, especially during a difficult conversation or when breaking bad news. Being flexible about allowing visitors to support the solo parent is a practical act of compassion.

Finally, show parents that you care too. While falling apart is not helpful, parents deeply appreciate feeling that their child is not just 'the baby in cubicle 4', but a real person, who is important and meaningful. While we're at it, it's a good moment to remind everyone that in general, child-first language is preferred. For a long time, healthcare staff have been discouraged from using condition or disease-first language. It is (in my humble opinion) grotesque to use phrases like 'the sickle cell patient' or 'the CF boy'. Many parents would rather focus on all the other things their child is, other than their condition.

How is all this relevant to breastfeeding you might ask? Well, when mothers are stressed and overwhelmed, this can affect their milk ejection reflex, and also their ability to be responsive. By caring for and communicating kindly with parents, you are helping to manage the inevitable stress they will be experiencing and supporting them to be calm, comforting and emotionally available to their child.

My top ten tips for communicating with parents

- **First of all, start from the assumption that parents are traumatised.** It's not normal to see your usually rambunctious and energetic child flattened by a disease. This can be traumatising. Trauma can manifest in many ways, but one of them is disassociation. This is a response by the mind to an event that is too stressful or traumatic to cope with. It is a way of disconnecting from reality. Many parents describe dissociation during part of their child's diagnosis, where they have large gaps in their memory, or feel apart from themselves. In fairness to health professionals, some parents may well put on a good act and appear to be having a two-way conversation, but if you start from the assumption that they are having a trauma response, this may mean that you protect the information you deliver by offering it in different forms – for instance, verbal and written, suggest they record a voice note so they can play it back later, and also repeat the information at different times, or to both parents.

- **Secondly, assume parents are exhausted and haven't slept.** They are also overwhelmed and parenting in a profoundly abnormal environment that is similar to a clinical goldfish bowl. There is no privacy, and it is extraordinarily stressful. At any moment, someone may knock on the door. It may be when they are getting dressed, having a private cry, trying to have a quiet argument on the phone, or on the toilet. Even if they are not traumatised, they are stressed and on high alert. It is highly likely that they haven't slept more than a few minutes at a time since their child became ill. The night staff may report that a parent has slept, but I guarantee, firstly – they may have only *looked* like they were asleep, and secondly, the time when they were 'spotted' sleeping may have just been a brief moment. Trust me, they are exhausted. It's not only tiring to not sleep, or achieve only poor quality sleep, but it's also emotionally exhausting to be worried about your child. Once they start to get better, it's unbelievably exhausting to try to entertain a child and keep their spirits up in this bizarre environment, far away from normality and their usual comforts, toys, favourite food and familiar things.

- **Thirdly, acknowledge and validate their medical expertise, if they have some, and their knowledge of their child's condition**, but then give them information that a ten-year-old could understand, and ask *them* to be the ones in charge of stopping you if you are telling them what they already know. Giving simple information is always best. It was Albert Einstein who said that if you can't explain it to a six-year-old, you probably don't understand it yourself. I absolutely believe this. Simple information may be something we think of as patronising, or belittling. This is nonsense. Some of the best lectures I have ever heard, by the best world leaders in a subject, have been brilliant not because of their unpronounceable words and unfathomable concepts, but because of their profound simplicity. I have found over and over again that one of the hallmarks of someone who understands something deeply, is that they are able to explain it simply.

- **Fourthly, never become desensitised to how big a deal it is to have a very sick child.** Never become so used to working with sickness that you forget that most people are used to and expect health and normality. Many health professionals are guilty of this, at least internally. Those 'bread and butter' conditions that make up the bulk of the general paediatric ward: the gastroenteritis bugs, acute exacerbation of asthma, febrile convulsion. Many health professionals do get a little institutionalised and can come to prefer something a bit more 'interesting'. But there are problems with this mentality. Primarily, nobody actually wants to be the parent of the child with an 'interesting' condition that is hard to figure out, and possibly hard to treat. Secondly, to the parent of the child with a 'boring' condition, the problem is unique, profound, and often frightening. We can sometimes become de-sensitised to the horror of these so-called common and 'boring' illnesses. Each and every hospital admission started with a sick child and a frightened parent, and we would do well to remember our humanity in that.

- **Fifthly, ask parents how much information they want at *this* moment, and whether it would be best to come back and give more information later.** Information is power. The right amount of information is like being handed the perfect manual and provided with one-to-one tuition. Conversely, too much information is like someone handing you three textbooks with no index and expecting you to digest it all alone. Assume that a parent needs the manual, but that they might need you to read them a chapter at a time, like an audiobook. They need you to also be the index, so that they can jump ahead and ask something that you haven't come to yet. If you know what you're talking about, this should not be a problem because you can mentally flip to that 'chapter' and deliver that information. What they don't need is for you to jump around on your agenda, giving lots of bits of information from all the chapters. The truth is, if you don't give people the information they need, their confused and traumatised brain will invent a scarier version of reality. There is no need to soften the truth – just deliver it softly.

- **Sixth, if you cannot speak to both parents, offer to come back** and give the information to the other parent (if there is one) when they visit, or write it down, ask the nurses to bleep the doctor to have a conversation on the phone with the other parent. Do not force a parent into the position where they not only have to absorb information but call it to mind and regurgitate it later on. This assumes that they remembered it correctly. I guarantee, they will only remember parts of it. Another helpful approach is for the child's named nurse to come with the doctor. Nurses are based on a specific ward, and have an allocated number of patients, while doctors work in teams, and have overall responsibility for a much larger number of patients. With the exception of a few clinical areas, most doctors are not based on the ward, but go around multiple areas to see all their patients, then begin to get down to the day's jobs, as well as cover the emergency department. They are much harder to get hold of, because by the time a parent realises they need clarification, the doctor may be stuck somewhere else with another pressing and urgent problem to attend to. Having a nurse present means they know what has been said and can reiterate the plan. If an interpreter is required, make sure both parents are around, and ensure that written information is provided as a back-up as well. If confusion is bad in your own language, imagine how much more frightening it is when you don't even speak the same language.

- **Seventh, ask parents if there is anything that still doesn't make sense.** Ask them what they are tempted to google later, and then address those areas of uncertainty to prevent random googling. As health professionals, it's easy to assume we've done a great job of explaining something, but I'd like to challenge people to assume the opposite. Assume that you may have left bits out, glossed over something, or not had quite the right explanation for this particular parent. Working from the assumption that we are not perfect is hard for anyone but by doing so will mean that you actively look for ways to help understanding. It means you are seeking an opportunity to better meet the needs of your patient's family. And asking them what they might google later makes you sound like a human who 'gets it'. It says to a family *'hey, this is scary as hell, but rather than type this stuff into a search* *engine later and get a million dodgy hits, I really am available right now to help you understand this. You don't have to wade into the murky depths of the internet'.* It also subtly acknowledges that you know you're not perfect, and that you're approachable. Trust me, you'll be loved for it.

- **Eighth, never assume a parent does not have issues of their own.** Clearly, the child is the patient, but parents are not always completely ok either. They may be sick, depressed, anxious, going through major life, relational or work upheavals. They may have financial strains, have a lot on their work plate right now, or have issues with other children they are concerned about. They may be neurodiverse. They may have learning or understanding problems. Always check their understanding, and always assume that there are other things going on in the life of this parent, who just happens to be related to your patient. Parents do not walk into the emergency department, ward, HDU or PICU as blank slates, committed only to the recovery and wellbeing of their child. They are frayed, broken, tired and dealing with other stuff that doesn't just go on hold because their kid is sick. They're worried about their child first and foremost. But they might also be worried about their cat, their job, their other kids, the rotting vegetables in the fridge, the builder who is supposed to come over tomorrow to look at the dodgy wall, and the car that's booked in for its MOT. Illness never checks to see whether it's a good time. It just arrives. The problem is, parents cannot put all the other stuff on hold, and they arrive with this baggage which adds to their mental load and anxiety over their child. Be patient with them. None of us knows what another human is dealing with in private. It's always best to assume there's a truck load of heaviness in the background.

- **Ninth, retain humility.** The most incredibly intelligent and learned people I have ever met have also been the humblest. Arrogance is false confidence and does not reassure. I cannot tell you how many times I have been most impressed by the people who have the humility to say, 'I'm sorry, I just don't know, but I'm going to have a hunt around, ask some people I respect, and come back to you.' It's been my experience that the more someone knows about a subject, the more they realise their own fallibility. It was Aristotle who first said, *'The more you know, the* *more you know you don't know'.* When you stay humble, you stay human.

- **And finally, show parents that you care too.** It's not helpful to dissolve into tears, but being human and showing compassion helps. To a parent, their child being sick is literally the worst thing they can think of. While we don't expect a health professional to jump into the pit of despair with us, we need to know our child is not just a statistic, a diagnosis, or a cubicle number. Showing that you care can happen in a myriad number of ways. Eye contact. An empathic touch on the hand. Simply saying *'I'm sorry you're going through this - it sucks'.* Asking how a child is, rather than assuming that you know by looking at the charts. It's also hard to succinctly summarise but caring about a child also means caring about their special adults too. FCC is at the heart of paediatrics and assumes the parents as experts and partners in care. But beyond that, it means caring for, looking out for and supporting parents too.

Maximising sleep

The final aspect of caring for families I want to touch on is the importance of maximising sleep. The occasional disrupted night can be borne by most people, and especially when children are sick, it's one of the inevitable aspects of parenting. But when a child is in hospital for more than one or two days, sleep deprivation can start to be really debilitating. The problem is that it's not just the disruption caused by a child waking or needing more comfort. It's also the hospital environment that doesn't lend itself to rest. Interruptions at night, noises, machines and interventions all cause additional sleep disruption which, after a while, can feel intolerable. Let's not forget that parents may arrive on the ward with their own physical / mental health or sleep challenges. Many adults suffer with insomnia, anxiety, sleep pathology or struggle with sleep due to (peri) menopause and not everyone is able to quickly return to sleep, especially in a high-stress environment. As I know all too well from my work with children's sleep, in general, parents of children under the age of three are going to be tired, because most children wake at night into their second year and beyond (Hysing et al, 2014).

So, start by questioning whether something absolutely has to be done at night. Could it wait until the morning? Of course, sometimes interventions, medication, treatment or monitoring is clinically essential, but anything that is not strictly necessary could potentially wait. If a child is clinically stable, routine tasks can wait to maximise sleep and rest for everyone.

If you have any control over the selection of furniture in your ward, consider the parent overnight beds. I have spoken with many parents who have found the beds that convert to chairs exceptionally uncomfortable. While most people can tolerate a poor night's sleep occasionally for a one-off hospital admission, I do feel particularly concerned for the parents whose children are resident on the ward for several days, weeks or months. The chair bed style parent beds are very narrow, which makes breastfeeding lying down difficult, as there simply isn't enough room for many parent-child pairs. It is also difficult if children prefer to feed with their mother sitting up. This means that unless there is a separate chair available, the bed needs to be converted back to a chair for feeding. Ideally, chairs that are comfortable for feeding should be provided *in addition* to the beds for parents. While I'm on this topic, I have heard many parents complaining that in open bays, the parent beds were all put away after breakfast. I've witnessed nurses militantly packing away all the beds as early as 8am in a behaviour that harks back to the old days of the matron inspecting everyone's hospital corners and ensuring the ward is tidy before the ward round. It's kind of archaic if you think about it, and not everyone is ready to start their day before 8am seven days a week (especially if they haven't slept - which frankly is likely when they are resident on a paediatric ward overnight with a sick child). This also makes it very hard for parents who normally feed lying down, feed their children to sleep, or indeed parents who take daytime naps. Could we be flexible? Could we make it clear to parents that they are free to clear their bed away, to create more space, or leave it out, as they prefer. Clearly there are some environments or clinical contexts where an unstable or deteriorating child may need prompt medical attention and a bed may be in the way. But this is not a universal scenario, and some flexibility and nuance is arguably appropriate.

I'll just share some practical interventions that I have either utilised myself or experienced first-hand as a parent from highly compassionate nurses who understood the importance of caring for parents in this way.

- Turn off alarms before entering cubicles or bays at night.
- If a bleep goes off, silence it promptly and move away from sleeping people to answer it.
- Make long phone calls in the ward office at night, rather than in open nurses' stations.
- Silence obs machines before checking children.
- Set alarms on your phone so that you arrive at an infusion pump *before* it alarms, ready with a flush to minimise disruption and noise.
- Set up noisy infusions, feeding pumps or syringe drivers outside of the cubicle or bed space, and then bring them to the child, ready to connect.
- Make sure children are proactively given adequate pain relief overnight to minimise discomfort.
- When children are hyper-hydrated for whatever reason, consider changing nappies or pull ups for a parent overnight, or collecting and emptying bedpans so they don't need to traipse to the utility room in the middle of the night.
- Even when parents usually give their child's NG feeds overnight, consider offering to do these for the parent so that they can get some respite sleep. Just because they are capable of doing all their child's usual cares, do not assume that this is not without sacrifice. Parents may insist on doing these caring activities for their child, but it is always compassionate to offer to assist.
- Minimise prescribing at night, so that, if at all possible, medications and IVs are given during waking hours, and only absolutely essential treatment occurs overnight.
- Avoid using bins with noisy lids in the night – take the rubbish back out with you. Even the soft-close bins can creak and disturb a light sleeper.
- And finally, facilitate bedsharing where appropriate to maximise sleep.

Bedsharing is fraught with complexity, controversy and complication. I have sadly known many parents to get shouted at, chastised and made to feel neglectful when they have told members of paediatric staff that their child usually bedshares. Of course, it is not always appropriate for a child to bedshare with their parent. However, bear in mind that if a child *usually* shares a bed with their parent at home, it is often not easy for them to sleep in a cot in hospital. In all likelihood, the options a parent is faced with are:

- Getting no sleep due to having to resettle and comfort their child in an unfamiliar sleeping environment at a time when they are already stressed.
- Sitting with their child upright in a chair all night, which we know is far riskier than sharing a bed.
- The child crying or being much more stressed for long periods, which will waste energy and reduce the amount of sleep they (and everyone in earshot) will achieve.
- The parent bringing their child into the parent bed, which is likely to be narrower, flimsier and will not have bed rails.

The pragmatic option for many families is to provide a child who is known to bedshare at home, with a full-sized bed, rather than a cot, and pull the bed rails up. Obviously, you will have to use your clinical judgement and risk-assess the situation for each family, but a full-sized single patient bed is usually much bigger than a pull-out parent bed, and is therefore much safer for bed sharing. Ultimately, if parents are used to bedsharing, they will conceal it or do it unsafely if they feel forced to do it for the benefit of the child. Given that the child is in a hospital environment and closely monitored, you may decide that on balance, given the alternative, this is a better option. If there is space in a room, it may also be possible to have a bed and a cot. The cot may be a useful safe place to have a child in the daytime when a parent is able to settle them for naps and rest, and then have the benefit of being able to bedshare at night. There are many good resources about bed sharing in the Appendix.

Deciding to stop breastfeeding

Finally, as well as supporting mothers to protect and maintain their milk supply, I believe it is also important to help them through ending their breastfeeding journey well. Sometimes mothers consider stopping breastfeeding altogether, either due to their child's condition, the contextual circumstances, or because they have had enough of pumping. They may also have reached their breastfeeding goal. How we stop is just as important as how we start.

What was clear from my first informal poll of mothers though, was that frequently the support was just not available, and recommendations to stop breastfeeding were often based on non evidence-based opinion, rather than true informed choice.

Before completely stopping, some mothers may appreciate considering their options. They may wish to donate their milk if they are stopping due to incompatibility problems such as PKU or chylothorax. They may wish to consider preserving their milk supply for a short time to see how the situation evolves. This may also be a good option to see how the infant tolerates formula, leaving the door open so to speak, in case the mother wishes to return to breastfeeding. Some mothers may feel that it is all or nothing and may not have fully considered the possibility of combination feeding.

Mothers who are stopping or reducing breastfeeding do require emotional and practical support, acknowledging and praising every day they have provided human milk to their child.

It is usually better not to stop suddenly, as this can be very uncomfortable and increase the risk of problems such as mastitis and pathological engorgement. Some mothers drop the equivalent of one feed or pump per day, every few days, so that stopping is very slow. Other mothers reduce the number of minutes they spend pumping each time, from say 30 minutes to 20, then 10, or extend the amount of time between pumping sessions, from three hours to four hours, and so on. Other mothers who are in a later stage of lactation may find that they can just hand express on an ad hoc basis to keep themselves feeling comfortable. It is always ok to express just enough to relieve the pressure. Milk production is driven by the degree of milk drainage, so as long as the mother is pumping or feeding less than they were before, their milk supply will reduce.

Mothers may also choose to use cold compresses to reduce inflammation, and they can also take anti-inflammatories.

Finally, particularly if the child was directly breastfed, the mother will need to provide alternative comfort measures to the child. This could be in the form of skin to skin with a non-lactating partner, as well as wearing the baby in a sling, cuddles, playing, and plenty of contact.

How stopping breastfeeding makes mothers feel

I genuinely believe that how we support mothers to stop breastfeeding is as important as how we support them to start or persevere. When reduction or cessation of breastfeeding is handled with compassion and enough information, mothers often describe feeling empowered and positive, rather than disappointed.

Even when the decision to stop or reduce breastfeeding is due to obstacles that are insurmountable in the face of their child's illness, this does not have to feel like failure for a mother if they are well supported. I have met numerous mothers who have breastfed previous children to natural term weaning, but due to an unsustainable pumping situation, fitting a complex feeding plan around their busy lives and perhaps other children, they make an informed decision to stop. Sometimes mothers describe their disappointment that they were unable to breastfeed their child in the way that they wanted or planned to, and yet they still feel that stopping was the right decision for them. Humans are capable of holding two or more complex and sometimes slightly contradictory emotions at the same time. They can be relieved that the round the clock expressing for a child who is not capable of orally feeding is over, and also sad that their child will never directly breastfeed.

The more we can have open and honest conversations with mothers about stopping, reducing or finding sustainability with feeding, the better their memory of breastfeeding or pumping will be. Sadly, I have also had many conversations with mothers who felt that stopping or reducing breastfeeding was something that happened *to them*, rather than them having a sense of ownership over it.

However breastfeeding is reduced or stopped, it is normal to have some mixed feelings about it. Some mothers decide to reduce

257

or wean because they are just ready or want to feel like they have their body back to themselves again. I have known numerous mothers who agonise over whether it is fair to deny their child the immunological properties and comfort of breast milk and breastfeeding particularly if they are very unwell. For these mothers it can feel a bit counterintuitive to place limits on a nurturing activity. If they are exclusively expressing, then they may still feel conflicted. Some mothers have found it helpful to consider:

- What is right for them, as well as their family. Continuing to breastfeed when a mother feels resentment or other negative feelings about it is not necessarily helpful. Breastfeeding is a relationship, and like all intimate relationships, it needs to have boundaries and be mutually agreed. If it feels com pletely one-sided, it may be time to consider some limits that help it to feel more comfortable.

- To what extent are the health aspects of breast milk affecting their decision-making? It may be helpful for a mother to be reminded that breastfeeding won't act as a panacea against all illnesses. It confers a normal rate of childhood illness. Feeling like breastfeeding will be the difference between health and illness, or life and death can be an enormously overwhelming responsibility that leaves mothers unable to make a balanced and informed decision.

- Many mothers feel they are being 'selfish' for stopping breastfeeding. Of course it is a decision that involves them and so by definition it is a decision that involves themselves. I remain unconvinced that this is *selfish* though. Mothers and parents matter too.

- Sometimes it helps to play devil's advocate. If a major reason for the reluctance to stop breastfeeding is due to the immunological components of breast milk, can they flip this around? How long would they have to breastfeed for until they feel fully guilt-free about stopping? Is that length of time sensible or achievable? If not, then logically, they will have to accept that they will be stopping before that time point. This may help them to make a decision that feels practical.

- Is it worth a compromise? Could they reduce to one or two feeds per day? The total 'dose' of immunoglobulins remains relatively constant, so as the volume of milk reduces, the concentration of immunoglobulins increases. This knowledge sometimes helps parents to come up with a plan to reduce that they feel more comfortable with.

There are many options for reducing breastfeeding (Hookway, 2021):

- Reduce the duration of feeds.
- Increase the interval between feeds.
- Intentionally distract to divert attention away from feeding.
- Offer an alternative to breastfeeding.
- Only consent to alternate feeds.

Sometimes mothers simply withhold the feed, and hold and cuddle their child, offering them reassurance and emotional support without feeding. Other times, this may be a non-issue if the child was not directly breastfeeding in the first place.

And if the mother is pumping:

- Increase the interval between pumping.
- Pump less volume each time.
- Reduce the total number of pumping sessions.
- Aim to reduce the total volume of milk pumped in 24 hours by a certain volume.
- Only pump at alternate intervals.

The comfort of the mother is important during an intentional reduction in milk volume. They may experience fullness or engorgement, depending on where they are in their lactation journey. Most people can take an over-the-counter anti-inflammatory, and many mothers find cool cloths and cold packs really soothing as well.

Finally, it's worth knowing that breastfeeding can help mothers return to sleep faster. Prolactin downregulates dopamine production. What happens when you stop breastfeeding is that dopamine levels start to rise again, which can make mothers feel really alert. They might find that it's harder to drop off to sleep than it was before. Anecdotally, I have also heard many mothers describing feeling low in mood or anxious when they stop breastfeeding, particularly if it is sudden. These effects are temporary, but mothers need to be able to make informed decisions. Mothers also frequently report feeling run down, and a pragmatic suggestion is for them to focus on eating well, drinking plenty of fluids, and taking a multivitamin. Many mothers also feel like this signifies the end of an era. It can help to acknowledge these feelings as normal. Mothers sometimes find writing a letter to their child about how they felt during this time cathartic, or they could keep a journal to remember this as a meaningful time.

The end of breastfeeding is in many ways inevitable, and positive, but it is not without some conflicting feelings and complex emotions. A professional who can understand the positive, negative *and* confusing emotions is one who will enable a mother to process these feelings most effectively.

Lactation after loss

It's a subject that nobody really wants to think about, but we do need to acknowledge that some babies and children die. Gillian Weaver first started talking about the 'milk of human sadness' many years ago and I'm grateful to her for a talk I attended many years ago. Sometimes a child's death is expected, and other times it is sudden. Either way, mothers who are lactating may have an additional layer of grief and complexity that we should be equipped to deal with (Cole, 2012). Recent research has suggested that a lack of anticipatory guidance about what will happen in terms of milk production can cause additional stress and be very upsetting (Marc-Aurele, 2020).

Mothers may not realise that they do have a range of options – broadly speaking these include suppression, expression and donation, and some mothers also wish to keep their milk as a memento.

The ongoing production of milk for a child who has died is a real and tangible link to their child, and mothers therefore may wish to give some thought to how to deal with their milk.

Of immediate concern is maternal comfort – they will need some compassionate support to keep their breasts comfortable. Breast binding is not recommended and usually just increases discomfort.

They can express for comfort or continue to express as per their previous pumping schedule, and may be able to donate this (Kennedy et al., 2107). It is often used for research, but may be able to be given to babies in need depending on the guidelines of the milk bank it is donated to. Other mothers have it turned into human milk jewellery, or some other memento. Some mothers just can't face making an immediate decision and maintain their pumping schedule until they feel ready to decide what to do more formally. Some mothers keep any stash of frozen milk in the freezer until they make a decision about what they will do with it – I have known mothers who have kept milk in the freezer for years as it remains a tangible link to their child. Other times mothers actively start to reduce the amount they express, extend the times between pumping sessions, or deliberately express less and less milk to gradually downregulate milk production.

Sometimes a more rapid reduction in milk production is desired. Sage is well known for reducing milk supply. Or you could consider pseudoephedrine. If you and the mother decide to choose the option of a prescription medication, cabergoline is the drug of choice, as it has fewer side effects than bromocriptine (Johnson et al, 2020).

It's important to think about what the mother might find triggering – for example, nursing bras, breast pads, a freezer stash of milk, and consider ways to manage the emotional pain of these memories.

There is support for parents provided by charities such as Child Bereavement UK, and The Good Grief Trust and plenty of training for professionals available from organisations such as the Stillbirth and Neonatal Death charity (SANDS) if you have not had much bereavement training. There are also a few helpful guidelines and frameworks to support practitioners who are helping mothers and families through this difficult time, such as the Lactation AID Framework (Carroll et al, 2020), so that you can provide practical support alongside bereavement care, including referring for psychological support.

Some immediate tips to handle this aspect of care compassionately:

- Use the child's name whenever you speak to the parents. Some people are concerned that to do so would upset the parents further. However, the worst thing imaginable has already happened – you cannot further add to their grief by speaking about their child, and in fact to avoid speaking about them may dehumanise the experience.

- If there is a member of staff that the parents had a particularly therapeutic relationship with, it may be best to refer to that professional. This is definitely not the time for the parents to be coping with a frayed or tense parent-professional dynamic which could just increase their discomfort.

- Allow parents to talk about their child as much or as little as they want to. Some parents will not want to talk about their lactation needs, but they do value someone listening to them talking about their child's life, illness or some aspect of care. Some parents also appreciate being asked questions about what their child was like, their favourite memory of them, or about their interests.

- Most people find being gentle, but matter of fact in their language helpful, particularly if there are siblings. Using phrases like 'gone to sleep' or 'passed away' are not always helpful to small children or people who struggle to decode figurative language. Simply saying 'I'm so sorry to hear that your child has died' is usually more helpful. Many people have also told me that they disliked hearing that their child 'lost their fight' as this implies that if they had perhaps been a little stronger they might have 'won'.

- Do not be afraid to ask gentle and supportive questions that may help the parents decide on the next practical steps. Asking 'do you need any information about how to manage your milk supply' allows them the opportunity to either explore that topic, or defer as they wish.

- Ensure that you have someone to debrief with. Particularly if you have had direct involvement in the care of the child who has died, this can take its toll on you emotionally as well.

Test yourself:

1. When a sick child is being breastfed alongside a sibling, which strategies would parents be likely to find supportive?

   a. Being flexible with visiting hours.

   b. Allowing both children to stay overnight.

   c. Offer some ideas for how to wean the older child.

   d. All except c.

2. Which of the following is an important aspect of FCC?

   a. Valuing the parents as partners in care and the experts on their child.

   b. Offering information in a few different ways.

   c. Offering siblings and parents psychological support.

   d All the above.

3. If mothers make the choice to stop breastfeeding, which is the *most* supportive action?

   a. Try to persuade them to carry on a little longer.

   b. Offer practical strategies and emotional support.

   c. Suggest a range of medications that might help.

   d. Suggest they leave the hospital for a few days so their child can't see them.

4. When a child dies, which of the following strategies is most supportive?

   a. Use the child's name.

   b. When the time is right, provide the mother a range of options for how to manage lactation.

   c. Offer the parent bereavement counselling if they wish.

   d. All the above

Chapter 11

Final thoughts

As we wrap up, I'll leave you with my ten top tips for supporting breastfed medically complex children.

1. Breastfeeding and expressing is not just about the milk. It provides a meaningful and significant form of comfort for both children and mothers, and promotes parenting self-efficacy and empowerment. We must value breast milk and breastfeeding as an important part of the child's holistic care.

2. Family centred care is not fully implemented in paediatrics/ PICU, and one of the areas where this is obvious is how breastfeeding is valued. The experiences of breastfeeding mothers need to be listened to - we must do better. This includes caring for parents better, so that their emotional, psychological and physical/health needs are treated as important. If parents require medical care while their children are inpatients, we need to find ways to make this happen to reduce illness, distress, anxiety and inconvenience to them. We must also treat families with respect and compassion, including providing culturally safe care, and asking about privacy without assumption.

3. Paediatric clinicians need to learn more about breastfeeding and lactation. But equally, nonclinical lactation supporters have gaps in knowledge that clinicians need to fill. We need each other. Collaborative, multidisciplinary working is the way forward. One way to address this is with joint training and jointly developed curriculums, as well as utilising those individuals with dual skills in paediatric challenges and lactation, such as our SLT/IBCLC, paediatrician/peer supporter, or paediatric nurse/ breastfeeding counsellor colleagues. These professionals have

unique insights into both areas of needs and challenges and can be extraordinarily helpful to achieve the nuance that is required. We also need to support our clinical colleagues who have lactation skills but do not come from a paediatric background, such as midwifery or health visiting, as they may be assumed to have the required knowledge and yet may need further training in the unique clinical challenges of older children.

4. We need to have ring-fenced funding for paediatric breastfeeding equipment, including designated breast pumps, sterilising equipment and specialised feeding devices - potentially at-breast supplementer and bridge devices. Ideally, we should also have a designated expressing room, with storage facilities for expressed breast milk. Additionally, we should be providing donor human milk as an option for children who would benefit from it, or when having to give formula causes distress and disempowerment.

5. Designated paediatric infant feeding teams should be funded to eliminate the skill deserts. These could include a combination of clinical and nonclinical lactation advocates who have all accessed specific training in supporting medically complex infants and children. A paediatric infant feeding lead should be appointed so that they can oversee the lactation needs of children on the paediatric wards and PICU, and not have to borrow expertise from other disciplines who may not be familiar with the challenges of infants and children beyond the neonatal period. The paediatric infant feeding lead should also be responsible for disseminating information and providing training, as well as leading on future BFI accreditation, audit and sustainability measures once the standards are truly established within the paediatric setting.

6. Specific training that caters to the needs of this population is urgently needed. It is not enough to transpose a combination of what works in maternity and neonatal settings. While some approaches and techniques can be 'borrowed' and adapted, some children have completely unique clinical scenarios and require a bespoke approach to adequately meet their needs. This will almost certainly require stakeholder input into educational competencies from nursing, medical, and allied health backgrounds that are specifically paediatric, rather than

neonatal or maternity focussed. The NMC, GMC and AHP educational competencies also need to be updated to include core competencies around infant oral feeding and supporting lactation.

7. We need nuanced feeding tools to become well-known and accessible on the paediatric ward, for example the feeding flock tools, as well as the assessment framework tool suggested in Chapter 8 and more nuanced tools that are fit for purpose - such as withdrawal scale tools that are designed for this population. We also need to provide anticipatory and proactive guidance for families for the next stage, whether that is stepped down care from PICU to HDU/general paediatric ward, or transitioning from enteral to oral feeding.

8. Furniture on the paediatric ward and PICU needs an overhaul. This includes both the physical provision of beds, chairs and pillows/cushions but also the approach to managing them. We need to remember that children sometimes breastfeed lying down, with their mother leaning back, during blood tests, straddling their mother's leg, or with large wounds. Children also sometimes breastfeed beyond the first two years, and chairs seem to have been designed with the assumption that only tiny babies breastfeed. Could we have a range of chairs available? Could we have some focus groups with breastfeeding mothers to ask which chairs would be most helpful? Could we make sure there is always a bed and a chair available? Could we provide bigger beds to facilitate safer and more practical bedsharing?

9. This is the most under-researched population within lactation. We may need to tolerate some trial and error and creative thinking when we encounter children with unusual challenges that test our clinical lactation skills. It's ok to ask trusted colleagues, come up with a working plan based on the advice and evidence we have, and then review it to establish whether that worked or not. When creative and unusual approaches *do* work, please can you write them up as case reports so that we can add to the sparse body of knowledge in this field?

10. And finally, we need to adopt a position of reframing breastfeeding as a normal part of caring for young children without age limits. Of huge importance is ensuring we do not have a 'formula default position'. Just because a child has severe laryngomalacia, we should not assume they cannot safely breastfeed. We should not write off children with certain conditions, or provide formula as the first solution when a child is intubated. This includes providing tailored and compassionate support to meet the needs of mothers and families, with the assumption that it is our job to facilitate families meeting their personal feeding goals. This means we may need to support mothers to continue to provide breast milk against the odds, return to direct breastfeeding, or stop breastfeeding in a respectful and appropriate way. Their goals, not ours, are what matters.

Where to go from here

We have reviewed the mechanism of infant feeding, both from the point of view of the mother and family, as well as the child, and how milk production works. We have explored why breastfeeding may be more difficult for medically complex children, and why it's worth persevering despite these challenges. We have also explored a range of ideas for supporting feeding in medically complex children, and how to make lactation and clinical care more family centred.

I wonder what you feel differently about? Perhaps you've been able to identify a need for more training in a particular area? Perhaps you could arrange to shadow a more experienced colleague or attend a breastfeeding clinic? One practical thing you could do straight away is find the breastfeeding policy, see who is responsible for updating it, and make sure it reflects current best practice. Then make it available; dust it down and place it in a prominent location.

At the present time, there are not many designated paediatric infant feeding leads, but you could network with your infant feeding lead colleagues in maternity and the neonatal unit to share expertise and resources. You could find out who the other breastfeeding champions are within your unit – you're unlikely to be the only one who is invested in making the environment more supportive for breastfeeding families. Then you could start to make the unit more overtly baby friendly – having displays, noticeboards, breastfeeding welcome signs, and support groups. These are all good ways to demonstrate that you are providing a welcome. Or could you go one step further and approach your manager, making a case to appoint a designated paediatric infant lead and team?

You could have some *'ask me about breastfeeding or expressing'* badges that those who are identified as having additional expertise can wear to help identify them to parents.

Ask for breastfeeding training to be mandatory for all patient facing staff, and challenge practice when you see or hear about poor advice.

Thank you for taking the time to consider the importance and value of breastfeeding for medically complex children and their families, and I wish you well as we all try to make the paediatric setting a more breastfeeding friendly environment.

Multiple Choice Quiz Answers

Chapter 2: How breastfeeding works

1. What triggers the onset of copious milk production?
   a. Frequent infant feeding.
   b. Domperidone.
   c. Genetic factors.
   d. The delivery of the placenta. (Correct)
2. What factors will downregulate milk production?
   a. Maternal fatigue.
   b. The degree of milk removal. (Correct)
   c. Having small breasts.
   d. Tandem feeding.
3. Breastfeeding is harder work for babies than bottle feeding.
   a. True/False. (False)

Chapter 3: Common breastfeeding challenges

1. What is a reliable sign of insufficient milk intake?
   a. Nipple pain.
   b. Jaundice.
   c. Cluster feeding.
   d. Poor weight gain and scant output. (Correct)
2. A mother exclusively breastfeeding her 4-week old infant presents with a fever over 39C, chills, tachycardia and a throbbing right breast. She has been on flucloxacillin for 48 hours with no improvement and feels acutely unwell. Which is the correct approach?:
   a. Advise the mother to go home, rest, drink fluids and take ibuprofen.
   b. Recommend immediate cessation of breastfeeding.
   c. Add in a second antibiotic such as co-amoxiclav and arrange to review her tomorrow.
   d. Arrange for hospital admission. (Correct)

3. Which of the following are risk factors for feeding challenges?

   a. Diabetic mother.

   b. Poor social support.

   c. Combination feeding.

   d. All the above. (Correct)

Chapter 4: Why feeding sick children is harder

1. Which factors related to infant illness may be associated with lactation difficulty?

   a. Inhibited milk ejection reflex.

   b. Lack of health care professional training.

   c. Needing to maintain milk supply.

   d. All of the above. (Correct)

2. Which of the following interventions is *most* supportive of lactation in medically complex children?

   a. Recommending that the staff bottle feed the child to give the parent some rest.

   b. Ensure mothers know that they don't have to breastfeed if they don't want to.

   c. Encourage skin to skin contact. (Correct)

   d. Explain that breast is best, especially when babies are sick.

3. Breastfeeding is not just about nutrition, but immunologic support, comfort and providing normality.

   a. True/False. (True)

4. Which of the following are valid reasons to breastfeed a medically complex child?

   a. It may be one of the few 'normal' parenting activities a parent can do.

   b. It provides comfort to the parent.

   c. It provides immunological support to the child.

   d. All the above. (Correct)

Chapter 5: Filling the gap in the current evidence base

1. Breastfeeding cessation is related to the severity of infant illness.
   a. True/False. (False)
2. Feeding assessments should consider which aspects of lactation?
   a. Maternal feeding goals.
   b. Infant age.
   c. What clinical procedures may interfere with feeding?
   d. All the above. (Correct)
3. Which of the following is supportive of breastfeeding?
   a. Asking how long a baby has been feeding.
   b. Telling a mother that they need to produce 90ml every 3 hours.
   c. Asking them how they feel feeding is going. (Correct)
   d. Suggesting that bottle feeding might be easier for them.
4. How should you use a feeding assessment tool?
   a. To highlight strengths and challenges.
   b. To reassure a parent that their child is ready to try feeding.
   c. To diagnose problems.
   d. All except c. (Correct)

Chapter 7: Keeping the milk going

1. Which of the following statements is NOT true about maintaining milk production with pumping?
   a. Pumping is easier for a mother. (Correct)
   b. At certain times, babies may not be able to directly breastfeed.
   c. Pumping/expressing is essential to maintain milk supply if a baby is unable to feed.
   d. Parents may need additional support and encouragement.
2. Which of the following strategies may support a mother who is struggling with an inhibited milk ejection reflex?
   a. Privacy.
   b. Relaxation techniques.

   c. Making donor milk an option to reduce the pressure.

   d. All the above. (Correct)

3. Which of the statements below is most supportive when working with a mother who is attempting to increase milk supply?

   a. Suggest that a mother asks their doctor for a prescription for domperidone.

   b. Encouraging the mother to drink 3 litres of water a day.

   c. Give them a rigid pumping schedule.

   d. Work with the mother to find a combination of pumping strategies that are sustainable. (Correct)

4. Which of the following is true of galactagogues and medications?

   a. Fenugreek is the safest galactagogue as it has been recommended for many years.

   b. All medications a mother takes will be found in trace amounts in human milk.

   c. Domperidone can be prescribed to all mothers whose prolactin levels are found to be low.

   d. Different mothers may need a different approach to increasing milk supply, and no drug or herb is necessarily safe for everyone. (Correct)

Chapter 8: When supplements and feeding pauses are medically necessary

1. Which of the following is NOT a medically necessary reason to supplement?

   a. Baby with Down syndrome. (Correct)

   b. Clinically significant dehydration.

   c. Hypoglycaemia that is unresponsive to optimised breastfeeding.

   d. Phenylketonuria.

2. Which of the following is a sensible reason to consider test weighing?

   a. When babies are fluid restricted.

   b. When babies are transitioning from tube to oral feeds.

    c. To reassure parents that their baby is feeding well.

    d. All the above. (Correct)

3. Which of the following methods of feeding is least likely to interfere with an infant's ability to breastfeed?

    a. Syringe feeding.

    b. Paced bottle feeding.

    c. At-breast supplementer. (Correct)

    d. Nasogastric tube feeding.

4. Regarding preoperative fasting times, which of the following is correct?

    a. Human milk has a slightly faster gastric emptying time than formula.

    b. There are national guidelines supporting the 4-hour pre-operative fasting rationale.

    c. Local policies regarding fasting times may vary.

    d. Both a and c are correct. (Correct)

Chapter 9: Supporting feeding in specific circumstances

1. For babies with low tone, which of the following strategies is NOT usually recommended?

    a. Dancer hand position.

    b. Upright feeding.

    c. Judicious use of a nipple shield.

    d. A 4-hourly feeding routine. (Correct)

2. Which babies are LEAST likely to become fatigued during feeding at the breast?

    a. Babies with Down syndrome.

    b. Babies with cardiac defects.

    c. Babies with cleft palate.

    d. Babies with phenylketonuria. (Correct)

3. Which strategies may support more efficient feeding?

    a. Breast compressions.

b. Frequent feeding.

c. Upright feeding.

d. All the above. (Correct)

4. When children are too sick to breastfeed, which is the *most* important aspect of care apart from ensuring the infant is adequately nourished?

a. Protect the maternal milk supply. (Correct)

b. Reassure the mother that they have done a great job.

c. Suggest the mother catch up on sleep.

d. Provide the mother with handouts on how to reduce milk supply.

Chapter 10: Emotional, practical and family-centred support

1. When a sick child is being breastfed alongside a sibling, which strategies would parents be likely to find supportive?

a. Being flexible with visiting hours.

b. Allowing both children to stay overnight.

c. Offer some ideas for how to wean the older child.

d. All except c. (Correct)

2. Which of the following is an important aspect of FCC?

a. Valuing the parents as partners in care and the experts on their child.

b. Offering information in a few different ways.

c. Offering siblings and parents psychological support.

d. All the above. (Correct)

3. If mothers make the choice to stop breastfeeding, which is the *most* supportive action?

a. Try to persuade them to carry on a little longer.

b. Offer practical strategies and emotional support. (Correct)

c. Suggest a range of medications that might help.

d. Suggest they leave the hospital for a few days so their child can't see them.

4. When a child dies, which of the following strategies is most supportive?

   a. Use the child's name.

   b. When the time is right, provide the mother a range of options for how to manage lactation.

   c. Offer the parent bereavement counselling if they wish.

   d. All the above. (Correct)

Appendix

Resources and FAQs for parents & professionals

If your child or patient has just been diagnosed with a medical condition, illness or disability, please start here. This is a collection of resources and guidelines. Note that research is currently *extremely* limited in relation to breastfeeding medically complex infants and children. As more information is available, it will be added. If you are aware of a useful resource, please contact me at lyndsey@ feedsleepbond.com

Many of these resources are UK based, but some are international.

Support groups

The Breastfeeding the Brave Facebook group is here: https://www.facebook.com/groups/358557901478129/

Beads of courage – charity acknowledging the bravery of children in adversity: https://www.beadsofcourage.org/

This website can try to link families facing the same condition up for peer support: https://www.cdc.gov/ncbddd/birthdefects/families-support.html

Short article I wrote summarising the evidence we have: https://www.all4birth.com/breastfeeding-medically-complex-babies-and-children/

Systematic review: https://onlinelibrary.wiley.com/doi/full/10.1111/mcn.13182

Guidelines and general information

The UNICEF UK Baby Friendly Initiative: https://www.unicef.org.uk/babyfriendly/

Breastfeeding course for paediatric nurses https://www.unicef.org.uk/babyfriendly/training/courses/a-course-for-paediatric-nurses/ and e-learning for paediatricians https://www.unicef.org.uk/babyfriendly/training/e-learning/e-learning-for-paediatricians/

My course, based on the material in this book: https://lyndseyhookway.com/product/breastfeeding-the-brave-one-day-course/

World Breastfeeding Trends Initiative. World Breastfeeding Trends Initiative (2020). State of Maternity Protection in 97 Countries: An analysis of WBTi country reports.

A Guide to Supporting Breastfeeding for the Medical Professional – book edited by Amy Brown and Wendy Jones

When Your Child is Sick – by Joanna Breyer

Your Child in the Hospital – Nancy Keene

Parental well-being

Being the parent of a sick or medically complex child can be challenging. Parents need to remember to take care of themselves. Here are some resources to help:

'For me as a parent' self-care activities (many of these can take place in hospital) http://formeasaparent.com/the-intervention-tools/self-care-activities/ and at https://parentselfcare.com/ and https://www.psychologytoday.com/us/blog/joyful-parenting/201708/25-simple-self-care-tools-parents. Headspace and Calm are good apps as well.

Formula and bottle feeding

First Steps Nutrition Trust – unbiased information about formula, including specialised formula: https://www.firststepsnutrition.org

Responsive bottle feeding from Baby Friendly: https://www.unicef.org.uk/babyfriendly/baby-friendly-resources/bottle-feeding-resources/infant-formula-responsive-bottle-feeding-guide-for-parents/

Financial and practical support

If you have life insurance with critical illness cover, it is well worth checking to see if you can make a claim on your insurance. This often applies even though your child is not named on your policy and will have no effect on your own cover.

Please also check with your social worker, or medical team.

Money advice service – providing resources about benefits and how to make a claim: https://www.moneyadviceservice.org.uk/en/articles/financial-support-if-you-or-your-child-has-a-disability

UK based support regarding government aided support: https://www.gov.uk/browse/childcare-parenting/financial-help-children

Also check with the hospital – they may have funds and grants to assist with parking, accommodation, and some charities provide a one-off grant.

Accommodation may be provided by the hospital, or there may be a home from home organisation near the hospital, if a child is cared for far from home. Try Ronald McDonald house: https://rmhc.org.uk

If friends ask what they can do to help, a meal train can take the hassle out of coordinating meals. Have a friend set this up and arrange the details for you: https://www.mealtrain.com

Pregnancy and birth

If you are pregnant and want to find out more about your options in labour and birth, in the first case, ask your midwife or obstetrician. If your child is diagnosed with a condition antenatally, you will probably be offered the opportunity to look around the neonatal unit. If not – please ask.

Here is some information from Bliss about how to prepare before birth: https://www.bliss.org.uk/parents/about-your-baby/before-birth

Birthrights website, about human rights in childbirth: https://www.birthrights.org.uk/

WRISK – understanding and communicating risk to parents in pregnancy: https://www.wrisk.org/

Infant Risk website: https://www.infantrisk.com/

Antenatal colostrum harvesting / antenatal hand expression information from La Leche League: https://www.laleche.org.uk/antenatal-expression-of-colostrum/

Expressing milk, and tube feeding

If your baby is born unwell, or becomes unwell, you will need to protect your milk supply by hand expressing and using a pump. Here are some resources to help

This is a video from Maya Bolman IBCLC: https://vimeo.com/65196007 about hand expressing and breast massage.

Parents may be using a breast pump on loan from hospital. If you need to source a breast pump, here are some (at the time of writing) WHO code-compliant ones:

https://www.ardobreastpumps.co.uk

https://www.hygeiahealth.com

https://www.ameda.com

https://www.limerickinc.com

https://pumpinpal.com

And some general information about pumping, including flange fit here: https://www.laleche.org.uk/expressing-your-milk/ and skin to skin: https://www.unicef.org.uk/babyfriendly/baby-friendly-resources/implementing-standards-resources/skin-to-skin-contact/.

You can read the WHO code here: https://www.who.int/nutrition/publications/code_english.pdf

This video by Jane Morton MD (http://med.stanford.edu/newborns/professional-education/breastfeeding/maximizing-milk-production.html) and also this website: https://firstdroplets.com/ which also has information available in Spanish about how to maximise milk production by using hand expressing as well as pumping, and power pumping information: https://themilkmeg.com/power-pump-your-way-to-more-milk/ and https://kellymom.com/hot-topics/pumping_decrease/

Some information and support here about exclusive pumping from Kellymom: https://kellymom.com/mother2mother/exclusive-pumping/

Some information here about using a nasogastric (NG) tube: https://www.gosh.nhs.uk/teenagers/your-condition/tests-and-treatments/nasogastric-ng-tube-feeding

Some information about using a gastrostomy (G tube):

https://www.cps.ca/en/documents/position/gastrostomy-tube-feeding

https://www.feedingtubeawareness.org/g-tube/

https://www.gosh.nhs.uk/conditions-and-treatments/procedures-and-treatments/living-gastrostomy-feeding-device/

You can read more about supplemental nursing systems, at-breast supplementers and the Laally bridge at these websites:

https://www.medela.com/breastfeeding-professionals/products/feeding/supplemental-nursing-system

https://www.lact-aid.com/

https://laally.com/

Re-lactation

If you are supporting a parent who is re-lactating, then in addition to the resources on increasing milk supply in this book, you may find the following helpful:

The Goldman-Newfarb protocol:

https://www.asklenore.info/breastfeeding/induced_lactation/protocols4print.shtml

The ABM protocol for LGBTQ parents has a large section on induced lactation:

https://www.bfmed.org/assets/DOCUMENTS/PROTOCOLS/Protocol%20%2333%20-%20English%20Translation.pdf

The ABM protocol for galactagogue use:

https://www.bfmed.org/assets/DOCUMENTS/PROTOCOLS/9-galactogogues-protocol-english.pdf

Breastfeeding without Birthing, by Alyssa Schnell (book) and breastfeedingwithoutbirthing.com

Donor milk, milk banking and drugs in breast milk

If a baby needs to be supplemented, check whether using donor human milk is an option. There are national milk banking organisations, and many hospitals have a milk bank on site.

The UK Association of Milk Banking (http://www.ukamb.org/) provides resources and information about the national milk banks in the UK.

Hearts Milk Bank (https://heartsmilkbank.org/) researches breast milk and provides screened donor milk to babies in need.

This is the Human Milk Banking Association of North America: https://www.hmbana.org/ providing information and links to milk banks across North America and Canada.

If you have a patient who is on medication and need to check breastfeeding compatibility, check out the Breastfeeding Network drugs factsheets https://www.breastfeedingnetwork.org.uk/detailed-information/drugs-in-breastmilk/, contact https://www.breastfeedingnetwork.org.uk/contact-us/, see the Lactmed website https://www.ncbi.nlm.nih.gov/books/NBK501922/?report=classic or visit the UK Drugs in Lactation Advisory Service https://www.sps.nhs.uk/articles/ukdilas/

Bed-sharing

Bed-sharing is a contentious subject, but it is known to facilitate more rest, and longer durations of breastfeeding. Different countries have slightly different guidelines and SIDS rates, which influences decision making and advice-giving at a policy level. There may be some children with medical complexity for whom bed-sharing may present additional risks, so an individualised risk assessment is appropriate. However, we must bear in mind that if bed-sharing is the norm for a family, and it is not facilitated in hospital, parents may find other ways of sharing sleep with their child that are less planned, and more unsafe. Here are some resources to read more:

https://www.llli.org/breastfeeding-info/sleep-bedshare/

https://www.basisonline.org.uk/parents-bed/

https://kellymom.com/parenting/nighttime/cosleeping/

https://www.lullabytrust.org.uk/safer-sleep-advice/co-sleeping/

Charities

Several charities will support parents:

https://www.sickchildrenstrust.org

https://www.macmillan.org.uk

https://www.younglivesvscancer.org.uk/what-we-do/

https://www.make-a-wish.org.uk

https://www.starlight.org.uk

Condition-specific support and information

Condition	Resources
Academy of Breastfeeding Medicine protocols	Includes protocols for cleft lip, pre-operative fasting, allergy, analgesia, diabetes and hypotonia https://www.bfmed.org/protocols
Arthritis (including JIA and JRA)	https://www.cdc.gov/arthritis/basics/childhood.htm https://www.arthritis.org/diseases/juvenile-arthritis https://cks.nice.org.uk/acute-childhood-limp https://www.cochranelibrary.com/cdsr/doi/10.1002/14651858.CD002824.pub2/full
Asthma	https://www.blf.org.uk/support-for-you/asthma-in-children https://www.asthma.org.uk/advice/child/diagnosis/ https://cks.nice.org.uk/asthma#!scenario

Condition	Resources
Autism	https://www.autism.org.uk/about/diagnosis/children.aspx https://www.childautism.org.uk/ https://cks.nice.org.uk/autism-in-children
Brain injury	https://childbraininjurytrust.org.uk/ https://www.braininjurygroup.co.uk/living-with-brain-injury/children-brain-injury/ https://www.headway.org.uk/about-brain-injury/further-information/useful-organisations/children-and-young-people/ https://www.braininjuryhub.co.uk/
Cancer	https://www.cclg.org.uk/childhood-cancer https://www.cancer.org/cancer/cancer-in-children/types-of-childhood-cancers.html https://www.cancer.gov/types/childhood-cancers
Cerebral Palsy	https://www.cerebralpalsy.org.uk/ https://raisingchildren.net.au/disability/guide-to-disabilities/assessment-diagnosis/cerebral-palsy https://www.nice.org.uk/guidance/ng62
Cleft lip/palate	https://www.clapa.com/what-is-cleft-lip-palate/ https://www.gosh.nhs.uk/conditions-and-treatments/conditions-we-treat/cleft-lip-and-palate https://www.clapa.com/treatment/feeding/breastfeeding/ https://www.laleche.org.uk/breastfeeding-a-baby-with-cleft-lip-and-palate/

Condition	Resources
Congenital diaphragmatic hernia	https://www.gov.uk/government/publications/cdh-description-in-brief/congenital-diaphragmatic-hernia-cdh-information-for-parents https://patient.info/doctor/congenital-diaphragmatic-hernia https://rarediseases.info.nih.gov/diseases/1481/congenital-diaphragmatic-hernia
Congenital heart defect	https://www.bhf.org.uk/informationsupport/conditions/congenital-heart-disease https://www.mayoclinic.org/diseases-conditions/congenital-heart-defects-children/symptoms-causes/syc-20350074 https://www.heart.org/en/health-topics/congenital-heart-defects/care-and-treatment-for-congenital-heart-defects/feeding-tips-for-your-baby-with-chd
Cystic fibrosis	https://www.cysticfibrosis.org.uk/what-is-cystic-fibrosis https://www.blf.org.uk/support-for-you/cystic-fibrosis/what-is-it https://patient.info/chest-lungs/cystic-fibrosis-leaflet https://www.marchofdimes.org/complications/cystic-fibrosis-and-your-baby.aspx https://jamanetwork.com/journals/jamapediatrics/article-abstract/515379
Diabetes	https://www.diabetes.org.uk/Guide-to-diabetes/Your-child-and-diabetes https://www.nice.org.uk/guidance/ng18 https://kellymom.com/health/baby-health/breastfeeding-type-1-diabetes-child/

Condition	Resources
Down Syndrome	https://www.ndss.org/about-down-syndrome/down-syndrome/ https://www.downs-syndrome.org.uk/ https://www.nhs.uk/conditions/downs-syndrome/how-to-help-children-and-young-people/ https://www.breastfeedingnetwork.org.uk/downs-syndrome-and-breastfeeding/ https://www.ndsccenter.org/wp-content/uploads/CDSS_breastfeeding_brochure.pdf
Epilepsy	https://www.epilepsysociety.org.uk/epilepsy-childhood https://www.epilepsy.org.uk/info/children https://www.gosh.nhs.uk/conditions-and-treatments/conditions-we-treat/epilepsy https://www.nice.org.uk/Guidance/QS27
FPIES	https://www.fpiesuk.org/ https://www.kidswithfoodallergies.org/food-protein-induced-enterocolitis-syndrome-fpies.aspx https://fpiesfoundation.org/about-fpies-3/
Gastroschisis, short gut syndrome and Exomphalos	https://www.gosh.nhs.uk/conditions-and-treatments/conditions-we-treat/gastroschisis https://www.cdc.gov/ncbddd/birthdefects/gastroschisis.html https://rarediseases.info.nih.gov/diseases/8661/gastroschisis https://www.gosh.nhs.uk/conditions-and-treatments/conditions-we-treat/exomphalos https://www.gov.uk/government/publications/exomphalos-description-in-brief https://www.niddk.nih.gov/health-information/digestive-diseases/short-bowel-syndrome

Condition	Resources
GORD	https://cks.nice.org.uk/gord-in-children#!scenario https://www.guidelines.co.uk/gastrointestinal/nice-gord-in-children-guideline/252583.article http://lifib.org.uk/reflux-in-infants-for-parents-and-carers/ https://www.breastfeedingnetwork.org.uk/reflux/ https://gpifn.org.uk/reflux-and-gord/
Hirschsprung's Disease	https://www.gosh.nhs.uk/conditions-and-treatments/conditions-we-treat/hirschsprungs-disease https://patient.info/digestive-health/constipation/hirschsprungs-disease https://www.niddk.nih.gov/health-information/digestive-diseases/hirschsprung-disease
Laryngomalacia	https://rarediseases.info.nih.gov/diseases/6865/laryngomalacia https://bestpractice.bmj.com/topics/en-gb/754 https://www.thoracic.org/patients/patient-resources/resources/laryngomalacia.pdf
Liver disease	https://childliverdisease.org/ https://childliverdisease.org/yellow-alert/ https://www.niddk.nih.gov/health-information/liver-disease/biliary-atresia https://kidshealth.org/en/parents/liver-transplant.html
Phenylketonuria and metabolic diseases	https://ghr.nlm.nih.gov/condition/phenylketonuria https://www.rch.org.au/clinicalguide/guideline_index/Metabolic_disorders/ https://www.ncbi.nlm.nih.gov/pmc/articles/PMC3383634/ https://www.jognn.org/article/S0884-2175(15)35340-5/pdf

Condition	Resources
Prader Willi Syndrome	https://ghr.nlm.nih.gov/condition/prader-willi-syndrome https://rarediseases.info.nih.gov/diseases/5575/prader-willi-syndrome https://www.pwsavic.org.au/get-support/early-years/diet-and-nutrition/ https://www.thealphaparent.com/triumphant-tuesday-breastfeeding-baby-6/
Sickle Cell Anaemia and Thalassaemia	https://www.sicklecellsociety.org/resource/sickle-cell-anaemia/ https://cks.nice.org.uk/sickle-cell-disease https://www.chp.edu/our-services/cancer/conditions/sickle-cell/resources/infants-and-toddlers
Skin conditions	https://www.dermnetnz.org/topics/skin-conditions-in-children/ http://www.dermatologist.org.uk/skin-conditions.html https://nationaleczema.org/eczema/children/ https://www.gosh.nhs.uk/conditions-and-treatments/conditions-we-treat/eczema
Spina Bifida	https://www.shinecharity.org.uk/spina-bifida/spina-bifida https://www.cdc.gov/ncbddd/spinabifida/facts.html https://www.nrshealthcare.co.uk/articles/condition/spina-bifida
Taste and smell disorders (can occur in isolation or with chemotherapy)	https://ueaeprints.uea.ac.uk/id/eprint/50291/1/Chem_Senses_2014_Philpott_chemse_bju043.pdf https://www.hopkinsmedicine.org/health/conditions-and-diseases/smell-and-taste-disorders http://www.anosmiafoundation.com/disability.shtml https://www.nidcd.nih.gov/health/taste-disorders

Condition	Resources
Tracheoesophageal fistula and oesophageal atresia	https://rarediseases.info.nih.gov/ diseases/7792/tracheoesophageal-fistula https://bestpractice.bmj.com/topics/en-gb/760 https://www.clinicalguidelines.scot.nhs.uk/ ggc-paediatric-guidelines/ggc-guidelines/ neonatology/oesophageal-atresia-and-tracheo-oesophageal-fistula/

Reference List

Academy of Breastfeeding Medicine Protocol Committee. (2008). ABM clinical protocol# 6: Guideline on co-sleeping and breastfeeding. *Breastfeeding Medicine*, 3(1), 38-43.

Academy of Breastfeeding Medicine. (2012). ABM clinical protocol# 25: recommendations for preprocedural fasting for the breastfed infant: "NPO" guidelines. *Breastfeeding Medicine*, 7(3), 197-202.

Ames, K. E., Rennick, J. E., & Baillargeon, S. (2011). A qualitative interpretive study exploring parents' perception of the parental role in the paediatric intensive care unit. *Intensive and Critical Care Nursing*, 27(3), 143-150.

Amitay, E. L., & Keinan-Boker, L. (2015). Breastfeeding and childhood leukemia incidence: a meta-analysis and systematic review. *JAMA Pediatrics*, 169(6), e151025-e151025.

Astbury, L., Bennett, C., Pinnington, D. M., & Bei, B. (2022). Does breastfeeding influence sleep? A longitudinal study across the first two postpartum years. *Birth*.

Atkinson, M. A., Eisenbarth, G. S., & Michels, A. W. (2014). Type 1 diabetes. *The Lancet*, 383(9911), 69-82.

Avidan, A. Y. (2007). Introduction to clinical corners in sleep medicine. *Sleep Medicine*, 1(9), 95.

Ávila-Alzate, J. A., Gómez-Salgado, J., Romero-Martín, M., Martínez-Isasi, S., Navarro-Abal, Y., & Fernández-García, D. (2020). Assessment and treatment of the withdrawal syndrome in paediatric intensive care units: Systematic review. *Medicine*, 99(5).

Bai, D. L., Fong, D. Y. T., & Tarrant, M. (2015). Previous breastfeeding experience and duration of any and exclusive breastfeeding among multiparous mothers. *Birth*, 42(1), 70-77.

Banta-Wright, S. A., Kodadek, S. M., Houck, G. M., Steiner, R. D., & Knafl, K. A. (2015). Commitment to Breastfeeding in the Context of Phenylketonuria. *Journal of Obstetric, Gynecologic & Neonatal Nursing*, 44(6), 726-736.

Bartick, M. C., Jegier, B. J., Green, B. D., Schwarz, E. B., Reinhold, A. G., & Stuebe, A. M. (2017). Disparities in breastfeeding: impact on maternal and child health outcomes and costs. *The Journal of Pediatrics, 181*, 49-55.

Beck, A. F., Solan, L. G., Brunswick, S. A., Sauers-Ford, H., Simmons, J. M., Shah, S., ... & H2O Study Group. (2017). Socioeconomic status influences the toll paediatric hospitalisations take on families: a qualitative study. *BMJ Qual Saf, 26*(4), 304-311.

Beck, C. E., Witt, L., Albrecht, L., Winstroth, A. M., Lange, M., Dennhardt, N., ... & Sümpelmann, R. (2019). Ultrasound assessment of gastric emptying time in preterm infants: A prospective observational study. *European Journal of Anaesthesiology (EJA), 36*(6), 406-410.

Beghetti, I., Biagi, E., Martini, S., Brigidi, P., Corvaglia, L., & Aceti, A. (2019). Human milk's hidden gift: implications of the milk microbiome for preterm infants' health. *Nutrients, 11*(12), 2944.

Bélanger, L., Bussières, S., Rainville, F., Coulombe, M., & Desmartis, M. (2017). Hospital visiting policies–impacts on patients, families and staff: a review of the literature to inform decision making. *Journal of Hospital Administration, 6*(6), 51-62.

Berecz, B., Cyrille, M., Casselbrant, U., Oleksak, S., & Norholt, H. (2020). Carrying human infants–An evolutionary heritage. *Infant Behavior and Development, 60*, 101460.

Berens, P., Eglash, A., Malloy, M., Steube, A. M., & Academy of Breastfeeding Medicine. (2016). ABM clinical protocol# 26: persistent pain with breastfeeding. *Breastfeeding Medicine, 11*(2), 46-53.

Bergman, N. J., Ludwig, R. J., Westrup, B., & Welch, M. G. (2019). Nurturescience versus neuroscience: A case for rethinking perinatal mother–infant behaviors and relationship. *Birth Defects Research, 111*(15), 1110-1127.

Bernt, K., & Walker, W. A. (2001). Human milk and the response of intestinal epithelium to infection. *Bioactive Components of Human Milk*, 11-30.

Binns, C., & Lee, M. K. (2019). Public health impact of breastfeeding. In *Oxford Research Encyclopedia of Global Public Health*.

Blomqvist, Y. T., & Nyqvist, K. H. (2011). Swedish mothers' experience of continuous Kangaroo Mother Care. *Journal of Clinical Nursing*, 20(9-10), 1472-1480.

Bode, L. (2012). Human milk oligosaccharides: every baby needs a sugar mama. *Glycobiology*, 22(9), 1147-1162.

Bode, L. (2015). The functional biology of human milk oligosaccharides. *Early Human Development*, 91(11), 619-622.

Bonner, J. J., Vajjah, P., Abduljalil, K., Jamei, M., Rostami– Hodjegan, A., Tucker, G. T., & Johnson, T. N. (2015). Does age affect gastric emptying time? A model– based meta- analysis of data from premature neonates through to adults. *Biopharmaceutics & Drug Disposition*, 36(4), 245-257.

Borra, C., Iacovou, M., & Sevilla, A. (2015). New evidence on breastfeeding and postpartum depression: the importance of understanding women's intentions. *Maternal and Child Health Journal*, 19(4), 897-907.

Bowlby, J. (1960). Grief and mourning in infancy and early childhood. Psycho analytic Study of the Child 15: 9-52. Bowlby, J. 1969. Attachment and Loss, Vol. I.

Bowlby, J., Robertson, J., & Rosenbluth, D. (1952). A two-year-old goes to hospital. *The Psychoanalytic Study of the Child*, 7(1), 82-94.

Bramer, S., Boyle, R., Weaver, G., & Shenker, N. (2021). Use of donor human milk in nonhospitalized infants: An infant growth study. *Maternal & Child Nutrition*, 17(2), e13128.

Briere, C. E., Lucas, R., McGrath, J. M., Lussier, M., & Brownell, E. (2015). Establishing breastfeeding with the late preterm infant in the NICU. *Journal of Obstetric, Gynecologic & Neonatal Nursing*, 44(1), 102-113.

Brimdyr, K., Cadwell, K., Widström, A. M., Svensson, K., Neumann, M., Hart, E. A., ... & Phillips, R. (2015). The association between common labour drugs and suckling when skin-to-skin during the first hour after birth. *Birth*, 42(4), 319-328.

Brown, A. (2022). *The Compassion Code.* Thought Rebellion.

Brown, A. (2018). What do women lose if they are prevented from meeting their breastfeeding goals? *Clinical Lactation*, 9(4), 200-207.

Brown, A. (2019). *Why breastfeeding grief and trauma matter*. Pinter & Martin: London.

Brown, A., & Arnott, B. (2014). Breastfeeding duration and early parenting behaviour: the importance of an infant-led, responsive style. *PloS One, 9*(2), e83893.

Brown, A., & Jordan, S. (2013). Impact of birth complications on breastfeeding duration: an internet survey. *Journal of Advanced Nursing, 69*(4), 828-839.

Brown, A., & Shenker, N. (2022). Receiving screened donor human milk for their infant supports parental wellbeing: a mixed-methods study. *BMC Pregnancy and Childbirth, 22*(1), 1-16.

Bui, A., Long, C. J., Breitzka, R. L., & Wolovits, J. S. (2019). Evaluating the Use of Octreotide for Acquired Chylothorax in Pediatric Critically Ill Patients Following Cardiac Surgery. *The Journal of Pediatric Pharmacology and Therapeutics, 24*(5), 406-415.

Butler, A., Copnell, B., & Willetts, G. (2014). Family-centred care in the paediatric intensive care unit: an integrative review of the literature. *Journal of Clinical Nursing, 23*(15-16), 2086-2100.

Campbell, S. H., Lauwers, J., Mannel, R., Spencer, B. (Eds). (2018). Core curriculum for interdisciplinary lactation care. Lactation Education Accreditation and Approval Review Committee (LEAARC), Jones & Bartlett Learning, Burlington, MA.

Canning, A., Fairhurst, R., Chauhan, M., & Weir, K. A. (2020). Oral feeding for infants and children receiving nasal continuous positive airway pressure and high-flow nasal cannula respiratory supports: a survey of practice. *Dysphagia, 35*(3), 443-454.

Carroll, K., Noble-Carr, D., Sweeney, L., & Waldby, C. (2020). The "Lactation After Infant Death (AID) Framework": A Guide for Online Health Information Provision About Lactation After Stillbirth and Infant Death. *Journal of Human Lactation, 36*(3), 480-491.

Central Health Services Council (Great Britain). Committee on the Welfare of Children in Hospital, & Platt, S. H. (1959). *The Welfare of Children in Hospital*. HM Stationery Office.

Chang, Y. S., Li, K. M. C., Li, K. Y. C., Beake, S., Lok, K. Y. W., & Bick, D. (2021). Relatively speaking? Partners' and family members' views and experiences of supporting breastfeeding: a systematic review of qualitative evidence. *Philosophical Transactions of the Royal Society B, 376*(1827), 20200033.

Chantry, C. J., Dewey, K. G., Peerson, J. M., Wagner, E. A., & Nommsen-Rivers, L. A. (2014). In-hospital formula use increases early breastfeeding cessation among first-time mothers intending to exclusively breastfeed. *The Journal of Paediatrics, 164*(6), 1339-1345.

Charpak, N., Montealegre-Pomar, A., & Bohorquez, A. (2021). Systematic review and meta-analysis suggest that the duration of Kangaroo mother care has a direct impact on neonatal growth. *Acta Paediatrica, 110*(1), 45-59.

Chen, C. H., Wang, T. M., Chang, H. M., & Chi, C. S. (2000). The effect of breast-and bottle-feeding on oxygen saturation and body temperature in preterm infants. *Journal of Human Lactation, 16*(1), 21-27.

Chen, C., Yan, Y., Gao, X., Xiang, S., He, Q., Zeng, G., ... & Li, L. (2018). Influences of cesarean delivery on breastfeeding practices and duration: a prospective cohort study. *Journal of Human Lactation, 34*(3), 526-534.

Choo, Y. M., Springer, S., Yip, K. X., Kamar, A. A., Wong, E. H., Lee, S. W. H., & Lai, N. M. (2020). High versus low-dose conventional phototherapy for neonatal jaundice. *Cochrane Database of Systematic Reviews*, (4).

Clifford, J., & McIntyre, E. (2008). Who supports breastfeeding? *Breastfeeding Review, 16*(2), 9-19.

Cole, M. (2012). Lactation after perinatal, neonatal, or infant loss. *Clinical Lactation, 3*(3), 94-100.

Colson, S. D., Meek, J. H., & Hawdon, J. M. (2008). Optimal positions for the release of primitive neonatal reflexes stimulating breastfeeding. *Early Human Development, 84*(7), 441-449.

Concheiro-Guisan, A., Alonso-Clemente, S., Suarez-Albo, M., Duran-Fernandez Feijoo, C., Fiel-Ozores, A., & Fernandez-Lorenzo, J. R. (2019). The Practicality of Feeding Defatted Human Milk in the Treatment of Congenital Chylothorax. *Breastfeeding Medicine, 14*(9), 648-653.

Cordeira, J., & Rios, M. (2011). Weighing in the role of BDNF in the central control of eating behavior. *Molecular neurobiology, 44*(3), 441-448.

Cox, D. B., Owens, R. A., & Hartmann, P. E. (1996). Blood and milk prolactin and the rate of milk synthesis in women. *Experimental Physiology: Translation and Integration, 81*(6), 1007-1020.

Czosnykowska-Łukacka, M., Królak-Olejnik, B., & Orczyk-Pawiłowicz, M. (2018). Breast milk macronutrient components in prolonged lactation. *Nutrients, 10*(12), 1893.

Daly, S. E., Owens, R. A., & Hartmann, P. E. (1993). The short-term synthesis and infant-regulated removal of milk in lactating women. *Experimental Physiology: Translation and Integration, 78*(2), 209-220.

Darbyshire, P. (1994). Understanding caring through arts and humanities: A medical/nursing humanities approach to promoting alternative experiences of thinking and learning. *Journal of Advanced Nursing, 19*(5), 856-863.

den Hertog, J., van Leengoed, E., Kolk, F., van den Broek, L., Kramer, E., Bakker, E. J., ... & Benninga, M. A. (2012). The defecation pattern of healthy term infants up to the age of 3 months. *Archives of Disease in Childhood-Fetal and Neonatal Edition, 97*(6), F465-F470.

Dettwyler, K. A. (2004). When to wean: biological versus cultural perspectives. *Clinical Obstetrics and Gynaecology, 47*(3), 712-723.

Dewey, K. G., Finley, D. A., & Lönnerdal, B. (1984). Breast milk volume and composition during late lactation (7-20 months). *Journal of Pediatric Gastroenterology and Nutrition, 3*(5), 713-720.

Dinour, L. M. (2019). Speaking out on "breastfeeding" terminology: Recommendations for gender-inclusive language in research and reporting. *Breastfeeding Medicine, 14*(8), 523-532.

Doherty, A. M., Lodge, C. J., Dharmage, S. C., Dai, X., Bode, L., & Lowe, A. J. (2018). Human milk oligosaccharides and associations with immune-mediated disease and infection in childhood: a systematic review. *Frontiers in Pediatrics, 6*, 91.

Douglas, P., & Keogh, R. (2017). Gestalt breastfeeding: Helping mothers and infants optimize positional stability and intraoral breast tissue volume for effective, pain-free milk transfer. *Journal of Human Lactation, 33*(3), 509-518.

Dumpa, V., Kamity, R., Ferrara, L., Akerman, M., & Hanna, N. (2020). The effects of oral feeding while on nasal continuous positive airway pressure (NCPAP) in preterm infants. *Journal of Perinatology*, *40*(6), 909-915.

Edwards, S., Davis, A. M., Bruce, A., Mousa, H., Lyman, B., Cocjin, J., ... & Hyman, P. (2016). Caring for tube-fed children: a review of management, tube weaning, and emotional considerations. *Journal of Parenteral and Enteral Nutrition*, *40*(5), 616-622.

Eglash, A., Simon, L., & Academy of Breastfeeding Medicine. (2017). ABM clinical protocol# 8: human milk storage information for home use for full-term infants, Revised 2017. *Breastfeeding Medicine*, *12*(7), 390-395.

Ekström, A., & Nissen, E. (2006). A mother's feelings for her infant are strengthened by excellent breastfeeding counseling and continuity of care. *Pediatrics*, *118*(2), e309-e314.

Elder, M., Murphy, L., Notestine, S., & Weber, A. (2022). Realigning Expectations With Reality: A Case Study on Maternal Mental Health During a Difficult Breastfeeding Journey. *Journal of Human Lactation*, *38*(1), 190-196.

Fallon, V. M., Harrold, J. A., & Chisholm, A. (2019). The impact of the UK Baby Friendly Initiative on maternal and infant health outcomes: A mixed-methods systematic review. *Maternal & Child Nutrition*, *15*(3), e12778.

Falszewska, A., Dziechciarz, P., & Szajewska, H. (2017). Diagnostic accuracy of clinical dehydration scales in children. *European Journal of Pediatrics*, *176*(8), 1021-1026.

Feist, N., Berger, D., & Speer, C. P. (2000). Anti-endotoxin antibodies in human milk: Correlation with infection of the newborn. *Acta Paediatrica*, *89*(9), 1087-1092.

Felice, J. P., Geraghty, S. R., Quaglieri, C. W., Yamada, R., Wong, A. J., & Rasmussen, K. M. (2017). "Breastfeeding" but not at the breast: Mothers' descriptions of providing pumped human milk to their infants via other containers and caregivers. *Maternal & Child Nutrition*, *13*(3), e12425.

Ferrarello, D., Froh, E. B., Hinson, T. D., & Spatz, D. L. (2019). Nurses' views on using pasteurized donor human milk for hypoglycaemic term infants. *MCN: The American Journal of Maternal/Child Nursing*, 44(3), 157-163.

Flacking, R., Ewald, U., & Starrin, B. (2007). "I wanted to do a good job": experiences of 'becoming a mother' and breastfeeding in mothers of very preterm infants after discharge from a neonatal unit. *Social Science & Medicine*, 64(12), 2405-2416.

Flaherman, V. J., Maisels, M. J., & Academy of Breastfeeding Medicine. (2017). ABM Clinical Protocol# 22: Guidelines for management of jaundice in the breastfeeding infant 35 weeks or more of gestation—revised 2017. *Breastfeeding Medicine*, 12(5), 250-257.

Flaherman, V. J., Schaefer, E. W., Kuzniewicz, M. W., Li, S. X., Walsh, E. M., & Paul, I. M. (2015). Early weight loss nomograms for exclusively breastfed newborns. *Pediatrics*, 135(1), e16-e23.

Flaherman, V. J., Schaefer, E. W., Kuzniewicz, M. K., Li, S., Walsh, E., & Paul, I. M. (2017). New-born weight loss during birth hospitalization and breastfeeding outcomes through age 1 month. *Journal of Human Lactation*, 33(1), 225-230.

Foster, K., Young, A., Mitchell, R., Van, C., & Curtis, K. (2017). Experiences and needs of parents of critically injured children during the acute hospital phase: a qualitative investigation. *Injury*, 48(1), 114-120.

Fox, M., Siddarth, P., Oughli, H. A., Nguyen, S. A., Milillo, M. M., Aguilar, Y., ... & Lavretsky, H. (2021). Women who breastfeed exhibit cognitive benefits after age 50. *Evolution, Medicine, and Public Health*, 9(1), 322-331.

Franck, L. S., Wray, J., Gay, C., Dearmun, A. K., Lee, K., & Cooper, B. A. (2015). Predictors of parent post-traumatic stress symptoms after child hospitalization on general pediatric wards: a prospective cohort study. *International Journal of Nursing Studies*, 52(1), 10-21.

Gannoni, A. F., & Shute, R. H. (2010). Parental and child perspectives on adaptation to childhood chronic illness: A qualitative study. *Clinical Child Psychology and Psychiatry*, 15(1), 39-53.

Genna, C. W. (2016). *Supporting sucking skills in breastfeeding infants*. Jones & Bartlett Learning.

Gephart, S. M., Weller, M., & Gephart, S. (2014). Colostrum as oral immune therapy to promote neonatal health. *Advances in Neonatal Care*, 14(1), 44-51.

Giudicelli, M., Hassler, M., Blanc, J., Zakarian, C., & Tosello, B. (2020). Influence of intrapartum maternal fluids on weight loss in breastfed newborns. *The Journal of Maternal-Fetal & Neonatal Medicine*, 1-7.

Goldfarb, W. (1943). Infant rearing and problem behavior. *American Journal of Orthopsychiatry*, 13(2), 249.

Goldfield, E. C., Richardson, M. J., Lee, K. G., & Margetts, S. (2006). Coordination of sucking, swallowing, and breathing and oxygen saturation during early infant breast-feeding and bottle-feeding. *Pediatric Research*, 60(4), 450-455.

Goldman, A. S., Goldblum, R. M., Garza, C., Nichols, B. L., & Smith, E. O. (1983). Immunologic components in human milk during weaning. *Acta paediatrica Scandinavica*, 72(1), 133-134.

Grace, E., Hilditch, C., Gomersall, J., Collins, C. T., Rumbold, A., & Keir, A. K. (2021). Safety and efficacy of human milk-based fortifier in enterally fed preterm and/or low birthweight infants: a systematic review and meta-analysis. *Archives of Disease in Childhood-Fetal and Neonatal Edition*, 106(2), 137-142.

Gregory, C. (2018). Use of test weights for breastfeeding infants with congenital heart disease in a cardiac transitional care unit: a best practice implementation project. *JBI Evidence Synthesis*, 16(11), 2224-2245.

Greve, L. C., Wheeler, M. D., Green-Burgeson, D. K., & Zorn, E. M. (1994). Breast-feeding in the management of the newborn with phenylketonuria: a practical approach to dietary therapy. *Journal of the American Dietetic Association*, 94(3), 305-309.

Griffin, S., Watt, J., Wedekind, S., Bramer, S., Hazemi-Jebelli, Y., Boyle, R., ... & Shenker, N. S. (2022). Establishing a novel community-focussed lactation support service: a descriptive case series. *International Breastfeeding Journal*, 17(1), 1-8.

Griffiths, B., Riphagen, S., & Lillie, J. (2020). Management of severe bronchiolitis: Impact of NICE guidelines. *Archives of Disease in Childhood*, 105(5), 483-485.

Grossman, X., Chaudhuri, J. H., Feldman-Winter, L., & Merewood, A. (2012). Neonatal weight loss at a US Baby-Friendly Hospital. *Journal of the Academy of Nutrition and Dietetics, 112*(3), 410-413.

Gupta, A., Suri, S., Dadhich, J. P., Trejos, M., & Nalubanga, B. (2019). The world breastfeeding trends initiative: implementation of the global strategy for infant and young child feeding in 84 countries. *Journal of Public Health Policy, 40*(1), 35-65.

Hahn-Holbrook, J., Saxbe, D., Bixby, C., Steele, C., & Glynn, L. (2019). Human milk as "chrononutrition": implications for child health and development. *Pediatric Research, 85*(7), 936-942.

Haines, C., Walsh, B., Fletcher, M., & Davis, P. J. (2014). Chylothorax development in infants and children in the UK. *Archives of Disease in Childhood, 99*(8), 724-730.

Hajian, H., Soltani, M., Seyd Mohammadkhani, M., Sharifzadeh Kermani, M., Dehghani, N., Divdar, Z., & Moeindarbary, S. (2021). The Effect of Acupressure, Acupuncture and Massage Techniques on the Symptoms of Breast Engorgement and Increased Breast Milk Volume in Lactating Mothers: A Systematic Review. *International Journal of Pediatrics, 9*(2), 12939-12950.

Heys, M., Rajan, M., & Blair, M. (2017). Length of paediatric inpatient stay, socio-economic status and hospital configuration: a retrospective cohort study. *BMC Health Services Research, 17*(1), 1-12.

Hale, T. W., & Rowe, H. E. (2016). *Medications and Mothers' Milk 2017*. Springer Publishing Company.

Hammerman, C., & Kaplan, M. (1995). Oxygen saturation during and after feeding in healthy term infants. *Neonatology, 67*(2), 94-99.

Hamner, H. C., Beauregard, J. L., Li, R., Nelson, J. M., & Perrine, C. G. (2021). Meeting breastfeeding intentions differ by race/ethnicity, Infant and Toddler Feeding Practices Study-2. *Maternal & Child Nutrition, 17*(2), e13093.

Hanson, L. Å. (1961). Comparative immunological studies of the immune globulins of human milk and of blood serum. *International Archives of Allergy and Immunology, 18*(5), 241-267.

Harlow, H. F. (1949). The formation of learning sets. *Psychological Review, 56*(1), 51.

Harlow, H. F. (1958). The nature of love. *American Psychologist*, *13*(12), 673.

Harlow, H. F., & Zimmermann, R. R. (1959). Affectional response in the infant monkey: Orphaned baby monkeys develop a strong and persistent attachment to inanimate surrogate mothers. *Science*, *130*(3373), 421-432.

Haroon, S., Das, J. K., Salam, R. A., Imdad, A., & Bhutta, Z. A. (2013). Breastfeeding promotion interventions and breastfeeding practices: a systematic review. *BMC Public Health*, *13*(3), 1-18.

Harries, V., & Brown, A. (2017). The association between use of infant parenting books that promote strict routines, and maternal depression, self-efficacy, and parenting confidence. *Early Child Development and Care*.

Harrison, D., Reszel, J., Bueno, M., Sampson, M., Shah, V. S., Taddio, A., ... & Turner, L. (2016). Breastfeeding for procedural pain in infants beyond the neonatal period. *Cochrane Database of Systematic Reviews*, (10).

Hassiotou, F., & Hartmann, P. E. (2014). At the dawn of a new discovery: the potential of breast milk stem cells. *Advances in Nutrition*, *5*(6), 770-778.

Heilbronner, C., Roy, E., Hadchouel, A., Jebali, S., Smii, S., Masson, A., ... & Rigourd, V. (2017). Breastfeeding disruption during hospitalisation for bronchiolitis in children: a telephone survey. *BMJ Paediatrics Open*, *1*(1).

Hester, S. N., Hustead, D. S., Mackey, A. D., Singhal, A., & Marriage, B. J. (2012). Is the macronutrient intake of formula-fed infants greater than breast-fed infants in early infancy? *Journal of Nutrition and Metabolism*, *2012*.

Hill, C., Knafl, K. A., Docherty, S., & Santacroce, S. J. (2019). Parent perceptions of the impact of the Paediatric Intensive Care environment on delivery of family-centred care. *Intensive and Critical Care Nursing*, *50*, 88-94.

Hinde, K., & Lewis, Z. T. (2015). Mother's littlest helpers. *Science*, *348*(6242), 1427-1428.

Holla-Bhar, R., Iellamo, A., Gupta, A., Smith, J. P., & Dadhich, J. P. (2015). Investing in breastfeeding–the world breastfeeding costing initiative. *International Breastfeeding Journal*, 10(1), 1-12.

Hookway, L. (2016). An exploration of common infant behaviour misinterpretations that can lead to a perception of low milk supply. *Community Practitioner*, 28-31.

Hookway, L. (2020). Breastfeeding the Critically Unwell Child: A Call to Action. *Clinical Lactation*.

Hookway, L. (2021). Still Awake. Responsive Sleep Tools for Toddlers to Tweens. *Pinter & Martin:* London

Hookway, L. (2022). Using art to raise awareness of breastfed children with medical complexity. *International Breastfeeding Journal* 17, 47

Hookway, L., Lewis, J., & Brown, A. (2021). The challenges of medically complex breastfed children and their families: A systematic review. *Maternal & Child Nutrition*, e13182.

Hysing, M., Harvey, A. G., Torgersen, L., Ystrom, E., Reichborn-Kjennerud, T., & Sivertsen, B. (2014). Trajectories and predictors of nocturnal awakenings and sleep duration in infants. *Journal of Developmental & Behavioral Pediatrics*, 35(5), 309-316.

Infant Feeding Survey, (2012) Infant Feeding Survey – UK, 2010. Available at: https://digital.nhs.uk/data-and-information/publications/statistical/infant-feeding-survey/infant-feeding-survey-uk-2010

Ingram, J., Woolridge, M., & Greenwood, R. (2001). Breastfeeding: it is worth trying with the second baby. *The Lancet*, 358(9286), 986-987.

Ivany, A., LeBlanc, C., Grisdale, M., Maxwell, B., & Langley, J. M. (2016). Reducing infection transmission in the playroom: Balancing patient safety and family-centered care. *American Journal of Infection Control*, 44(1), 61-65.

Järvinen, K. M., Martin, H., & Oyoshi, M. K. (2019). Immunomodulatory Effects of Breast Milk on Food Allergy. *Annals of Allergy, Asthma & Immunology.*

Jensen, D., Wallace, S., & Kelsay, P. (1994). LATCH: a breastfeeding charting system and documentation tool. *Journal of Obstetric, Gynecologic, & Neonatal Nursing*, 23(1), 27-32.

Johnson, H. M., Eglash, A., Mitchell, K. B., Leeper, K., Smillie, C. M., Moore-Ostby, L., ... & Academy of Breastfeeding Medicine. (2020). ABM Clinical Protocol# 32: management of hyperlactation. *Breastfeeding Medicine, 15*(3), 129-134.

Johnston, C. C., Filion, F., Campbell-Yeo, M., Goulet, C., Bell, L., McNaughton, K., & Byron, J. (2009). Enhanced kangaroo mother care for heel lance in preterm neonates: a crossover trial. *Journal of Perinatology, 29*(1), 51-56.

Jones, W. (2018). *Breastfeeding and Medication*. Routledge.

Juncker, H. G., Romijn, M., Loth, V. N., Caniels, T. G., de Groot, C. J., Pajkrt, D., ... & van Keulen, B. J. (2021). Human Milk Antibodies Against SARS-CoV-2: A Longitudinal Follow-Up Study. *Journal of Human Lactation, 37*(3), 485-491.

Kair, L. R., & Flaherman, V. J. (2017). Donor milk or formula: a qualitative study of postpartum mothers of healthy newborns. *Journal of Human Lactation, 33*(4), 710-716.

Kantorowska, A., Wei, J. C., Cohen, R. S., Lawrence, R. A., Gould, J. B., & Lee, H. C. (2016). Impact of donor milk availability on breast milk use and necrotizing enterocolitis rates. *Pediatrics, 137*(3).

Karampatsas, K., Kong, J., & Cohen, J. (2019). Bronchiolitis: an update on management and prophylaxis. *British Journal of Hospital Medicine, 80*(5), 278-284.

Keeble, E., & Kossarova, L. (2017). Focus on: Emergency hospital care for children and young people. *Focus on Research Report. QualityWatch*.

Kelly, B. N., Huckabee, M. L., Jones, R. D., & Frampton, C. M. (2007). The First Year of Human Life: Coordinating Respiration and Nutritive Swallowing. *Dysphagia, 22*(1), 37.

Kendall-Tackett, K. (2015). The new paradigm for depression in new mothers: current findings on maternal depression, breastfeeding and resiliency across the lifespan. *Breastfeeding Review, 23*(1), 7-10.

Kennedy, J., Matthews, A., Abbott, L., Dent, J., Weaver, G., & Shenker, N. (2017). Lactation following bereavement: how can midwives support women to make informed choices? *MIDIRS Midwifery Digest*.

Kent, J. C., Hepworth, A. R., Langton, D. B., & Hartmann, P. E. (2015). Impact of measuring milk production by test weighing on breastfeeding confidence in mothers of term infants. *Breastfeeding Medicine*, 10(6), 318-325.

Kent, J. C., Hepworth, A. R., Sherriff, J. L., Cox, D. B., Mitoulas, L. R., & Hartmann, P. E. (2013). Longitudinal changes in breastfeeding patterns from 1 to 6 months of lactation. *Breastfeeding Medicine*, 8(4), 401-407.

Kent, J. C., Mitoulas, L. R., Cregan, M. D., Geddes, D. T., Larsson, M., Doherty, D. A., & Hartmann, P. E. (2008). Importance of vacuum for breastmilk expression. *Breastfeeding Medicine*, 3(1), 11-19.

Kish, A. M., Newcombe, P. A., & Haslam, D. M. (2018). Working and caring for a child with chronic illness: a review of current literature. *Child: Care, Health and Development*, 44(3), 343-354.

Koppen, I. J., Vriesman, M. H., Saps, M., Rajindrajith, S., Shi, X., van Etten-Jamaludin, F. S., ... & Tabbers, M. M. (2018). Prevalence of functional defecation disorders in children: a systematic review and meta-analysis. *The Journal of Pediatrics*, 198, 121-130.

Krüger et al. (2019). Oropharyngeal Dysphagia in Breastfeeding Neonates with Hypoxic-Ischemic Encephalopathy on Therapeutic Hypothermia. *Breastfeeding Medicine*, 14(10), 718-723.

Lackey, K. A., Fehrenkamp, B. D., Pace, R. M., Williams, J. E., Meehan, C. L., McGuire, M. A., & McGuire, M. K. (2021). Breastfeeding Beyond 12 Months: Is There Evidence for Health Impacts?. *Annual Review of Nutrition*, 283-308.

Laguna-Cruz, C. R., & Becina, G. T. (2017). Association Between Breastfeeding and Clinical Outcomes of Infants with Very Severe Pneumonia. *Pediatric Infectious Disease Society of the Philippines Journal*, 18 (1), 3-10.

Lambert, J. M., & Watters, N. E. (1998). Breastfeeding the infant/child with a cardiac defect: an informal survey. *Journal of Human Lactation*, 14(2), 151-155.

Lamberti, L. M., Zakarija-Grković, I., Fischer Walker, C. L., Theodoratou, E., Nair, H., Campbell, H., & Black, R. E. (2013). Breastfeeding for reducing the risk of pneumonia morbidity and mortality in children under two: a systematic literature review and meta-analysis. *BMC Public Health*, 13(3), 1-8.

Larson-Meyer, D. E., Schueler, J., Kyle, E., Austin, K. J., Hart, A. M., & Alexander, B. M. (2021). Appetite-regulating hormones in human milk: a plausible biological factor for obesity risk reduction?. *Journal of Human Lactation*, 37(3), 603-614.

Lawlor & Choi. (2020). Diagnosis and management of pediatric dysphagia: a review. *JAMA Otolaryngology–Head & Neck Surgery*, 146(2), 183-191.

Lawrence, R. M. (2022). Host-resistance factors and immunologic significance of human milk. In *Breastfeeding* (pp. 145-192). Elsevier.

LeFort, Y., Evans, A., Livingstone, V., Douglas, P., Dahlquist, N., Donnelly, B., ... & Academy of Breastfeeding Medicine. (2021). Academy of Breastfeeding Medicine Position Statement on ankyloglossia in breastfeeding dyads. *Breastfeeding Medicine*, 16(4), 278-281.

Lewis, E., & Kritzinger, A. (2004). Parental experiences of feeding problems in their infants with Down syndrome. *Down Syndrome Research and Practice*, 9(2), 45-52.

Little, E. E., Legare, C. H., & Carver, L. J. (2018). Mother–Infant physical contact predicts responsive feeding among US breastfeeding mothers. *Nutrients*, 10(9), 1251.

Lucas, R., Gupton, S., Holditch-Davis, D., & Brandon, D. (2014). A case study of a late preterm infant's transition to full at-breast feedings at 4 months of age. *Journal of Human Lactation*, 30(1), 28-30.

Madhoun, L. L., Crerand, C. E., Keim, S., & Baylis, A. L. (2020). Breast Milk Feeding Practices and Barriers and Supports Experienced by Mother–Infant Dyads with Cleft Lip and/or Palate. *The Cleft Palate-Craniofacial Journal*, 57(4), 477-486.

Malouf, R., Harrison, S., Burton, H. A., Gale, C., Stein, A., Franck, L. S., & Alderdice, F. (2022). Prevalence of anxiety and post-traumatic stress (PTS) among the parents of babies admitted to neonatal units: A systematic review and meta-analysis. *E Clinical Medicine*, 43, 101233.

Mangel, L., Mimouni, F. B., Mandel, D., Mordechaev, N., & Marom, R. (2019). Breastfeeding difficulties, breastfeeding duration, maternal Body Mass Index, and breast anatomy: Are they related? *Breastfeeding Medicine*, 14(5), 342-346.

Mangel, L., Ovental, A., Batscha, N., Arnon, M., Yarkoni, I., & Dollberg, S. (2015). Higher fat content in breastmilk expressed manually: a randomized trial. *Breastfeeding Medicine*, 10(7), 352-354.

Marc-Aurele, K. L. (2020). Decisions Parents Make When Faced with Potentially Life-Limiting Fetal Diagnoses and the Importance of Perinatal Palliative Care. *Frontiers in Pediatrics*, 8, 671.

Martin, H., van Wijngaarden, E., Seplaki, C. L., Stringer, J., Williams, G. C., & Dozier, A. M. (2021). Breastfeeding Motivation Predicts Infant Feeding Intention and Outcomes: Evaluation of a Novel Adaptation of the Treatment Self-Regulation Questionnaire. *Journal of Human Lactation*, 08903344211032128.

Marvin-Dowle, K., Soltani, H., & Spencer, R. (2021). Infant feeding in diverse families; the impact of ethnicity and migration on feeding practices. *Midwifery*, 103, 103124.

Mastandrea, S., Fagioli, S., & Biasi, V. (2019). Art and psychological well-being: Linking the brain to the aesthetic emotion. *Frontiers in Psychology*, 10, 739.

Matthews, M. K. (1988). Developing an instrument to assess infant breastfeeding behaviour in the early neonatal period. *Midwifery*, 4(4), 154-165.

Matthews, K., Webber, K., McKim, E., Banoub-Baddour, S., & Laryea, M. (1998). Maternal infant-feeding decisions: reasons and influences. *Canadian Journal of Nursing Research Archive*, 30(2).

McCue, K. F., & Stulberger, M. L. (2019). Maternal satisfaction with parallel pumping technique. *Clinical Lactation*, 10(2), 68-73.

McCune, S., & Perrin, M. T. (2021). Donor human milk use in populations other than the preterm infant: a systematic scoping review. *Breastfeeding Medicine*, 16(1), 8-20.

McFadden, A., Gavine, A., Renfrew, M. J., Wade, A., Buchanan, P., Taylor, J. L., ... & MacGillivray, S. (2017). Support for healthy breastfeeding mothers with healthy term babies. *Cochrane Database of Systematic Reviews*, (2).

McKenna, J. J., Ball, H. L., & Gettler, L. T. (2007). Mother–infant cosleeping, breastfeeding and sudden infant death syndrome: what biological anthropology has discovered about normal infant sleep and pediatric sleep medicine. *American Journal of Physical Anthropology: The Official Publication of the American Association of Physical Anthropologists, 134*(S45), 133-161.

McKenna, J. J., & Gettler, L. T. (2016). There is no such thing as infant sleep, there is no such thing as breastfeeding, there is only breastsleeping. *Acta Paediatrica, 105*(1), 17-21.

McLaughlin, M., Fraser, J., Young, J., & Keogh, S. (2011). Paediatric nurses' knowledge and attitudes related to breastfeeding and the hospitalised infant. *Breastfeeding Review, 19*(3), 13.

Medoff-Cooper, B., Naim, M., Torowicz, D., & Mott, A. (2010). Feeding, growth, and nutrition in children with congenitally malformed hearts. *Cardiology in the Young, 20*(S3), 149-153.

Menninghaus, W., Wagner, V., Hanich, J., Wassiliwizky, E., Jacobsen, T., & Koelsch, S. (2017). The Distancing-Embracing model of the enjoyment of negative emotions in art reception. *The Behavioral and Brain Sciences, 40*, e347.

Milinco, M., Travan, L., Cattaneo, A., Knowles, A., Sola, M. V., Causin, E., ... & Ronfani, L. (2020). Effectiveness of biological nurturing on early breastfeeding problems: a randomized controlled trial. *International Breastfeeding Journal, 15*(1), 1-10.

Miller, D., Mamilly, L., Fourtner, S., Rosen-Carole, C., & Academy of Breastfeeding Medicine. (2017). ABM Clinical Protocol# 27: breastfeeding an infant or young child with insulin-dependent diabetes. *Breastfeeding Medicine, 12*(2), 72-76.

Mitchell, K. B., Johnson, H. M., Eglash, A., & Academy of Breastfeeding Medicine. (2019). ABM clinical protocol# 30: breast masses, breast complaints, and diagnostic breast imaging in the lactating woman. *Breastfeeding Medicine, 14*(4), 208-214.

Mitchell, K. B., Johnson, H. M., Rodríguez, J. M., Eglash, A., Scherzinger, C., Zakarija-Grkovic, I., ... & Academy of Breastfeeding Medicine. (2022). Academy of Breastfeeding Medicine Clinical Protocol# 36: The Mastitis Spectrum, Revised 2022. *Breastfeeding Medicine, 17*(5), 360-376.

Mitchell, A. E., Morawska, A., & Mihelic, M. (2020). A systematic review of parenting interventions for child chronic health conditions. *Journal of Child Health Care, 24*(4), 603-628.

Mitting, R. B., Peshimam, N., Lillie, J., Donnelly, P., Ghazaly, M., Nadel, S., ... & Tibby, S. M. (2021). Invasive mechanical ventilation for acute viral bronchiolitis: retrospective multicenter cohort study. *Pediatric Critical Care Medicine*, 22(3), 231-240.

Moberg, K. U., & Prime, D. K. (2013). Oxytocin effects in mothers and infants during breastfeeding. *Infant*, 9(6), 201-206.

Moore, D. B., & Catlin, A. (2003). Lactation suppression: forgotten aspect of care for the mother of a dying child. *Pediatric Nursing*, 29(5), 383-4.

Moore, E. R., Bergman, N., Anderson, G. C., & Medley, N. (2016). Early skin-to-skin contact for mothers and their healthy newborn infants. *Cochrane Database of Systematic Reviews*, (11).

Moossavi, S., Sepehri, S., Robertson, B., Bode, L., Goruk, S., Field, C. J., ... & Azad, M. B. (2019). Composition and variation of the human milk microbiota are influenced by maternal and early-life factors. *Cell Host & Microbe*, 25(2), 324-335.

Morag, I., Hendel, Y., Karol, D., Geva, R., & Tzipi, S. (2019). Transition from Nasogastric Tube to Oral Feeding: The Role of Parental Guided Responsive Feeding. *Frontiers in Pediatrics*, 7, 190.

Moral, A., Bolibar, I., Seguranyes, G., Ustrell, J. M., Sebastiá, G., Martínez-Barba, C., & Ríos, J. (2010). Mechanics of sucking: comparison between bottle feeding and breastfeeding. *BMC Pediatrics*, 10(1), 1-8.

Mortensen, J., Simonsen, B. O., Eriksen, S. B., Skovby, P., Dall, R., & Elklit, A. (2015). Family-centred care and traumatic symptoms in parents of children admitted to PICU. *Scandinavian Journal of Caring Sciences*, 29(3), 495-500.

Morton, J. (2014). Perfect storm or perfect time for a bold change? *Breastfeeding Medicine*, 9(4), 180-183.

Morton, J., Hall, J. Y., Wong, R. J., Thairu, L., Benitz, W. E., & Rhine, W. D. (2009). Combining hand techniques with electric pumping increases milk production in mothers of preterm infants. *Journal of Perinatology*, 29(11), 757-764.

Morton, J., Wong, R. J., Hall, J. Y., Pang, W. W., Lai, C. T., Lui, J., ... & Rhine, W. D. (2012). Combining hand techniques with electric pumping increases the caloric content of milk in mothers of preterm infants. *Journal of Perinatology, 32*(10), 791-796.

Mulford, C. (1992). The mother-baby assessment (MBA): An" Apgar Score" for breastfeeding. *Journal of Human lactation, 8*(2), 79-82.

Murray, B. L., Kenardy, J. A., & Spence, S. H. (2007). Brief report: Children's responses to trauma-and nontrauma-related hospital admission: A comparison study. *Journal of Pediatric Psychology, 33*(4), 435-440.

Muscara, F., McCarthy, M. C., Woolf, C., Hearps, S. J. C., Burke, K., & Anderson, V. A. (2015). Early psychological reactions in parents of children with a life threatening illness within a pediatric hospital setting. *European Psychiatry, 30*(5), 555-561.

Narayanan et al. (1991). Sucking on the 'emptied' breast: non-nutritive sucking with a difference. *Archives of Disease in Childhood,* 66(2), 241-244.

National Collaborating Centre for Women's and Children's Health (UK. (2009). Diarrhoea and vomiting caused by gastroenteritis: diagnosis, assessment and management in children younger than 5 years.

Negin, J., Coffman, J., Vizintin, P., & Raynes-Greenow, C. (2016). The influence of grandmothers on breastfeeding rates: a systematic review. *BMC Pregnancy and Childbirth, 16*(1), 1-10.

Neill, S., Roland, D., Thompson, M., Tavaré, A., & Lakhanpaul, M. (2018). Why are acute admissions to hospital of children under 5 years of age increasing in the UK?. *Archives of Disease in Childhood,* 103(10), 917-919.

NICE Clinical Knowledge Summary on Faltering Growth, (2018) Available at: https://cks.nice.org.uk/topics/faltering-growth/diagnosis/assessment/#:~:text=The%20NICE%20guideline%20on%20faltering%20growth%20%5B%20NICE%2C,to%20help%20inform%20management%20strategies%20and%20assess%-20progress.

NICE Clinical Knowledge Summary on Bronchiolitis in children: diagnosis and management (2015) Available at: https://www.nice.org.uk/guidance/ng9

Nimmo, S. (2019). Please don't call me mum. *BMJ*, *367*.

Noble, L. M., Okogbule-Wonodi, A. C., Young, M. A., & Academy of Breastfeeding Medicine. (2018). ABM Clinical Protocol# 12: Transitioning the breastfeeding preterm infant from the neonatal intensive care unit to home, revised 2018. *Breastfeeding Medicine*, *13*(4), 230-236.

Noel-Weiss, J., Courant, G., & Woodend, A. K. (2008). Physiological weight loss in the breastfed neonate: a systematic review. *Open Medicine*, *2*(4), e99.

Nyqvist, K. H., & Ewald, U. (1999). Infant and maternal factors in the development of breastfeeding behaviour and breastfeeding outcome in preterm infants. *Acta Paediatrica*, *88*(11), 1194-1203.

Oakley, E., Borland, M., Neutze, J., Acworth, J., Krieser, D., Dalziel, S., ... & Paediatric Research in Emergency Departments International Collaborative (PREDICT. (2013). Nasogastric hydration versus intravenous hydration for infants with bronchiolitis: a randomised trial. *The Lancet Respiratory Medicine*, *1*(2), 113-120.

Ongkasuwan & Chiou. (2018). Paediatric Dysphagia: Challenges and Controversies. Springer Nature, Switzerland.

Pados, B. F., Estrem, H. H., Thoyre, S. M., Park, J., & McComish, C. (2017). The neonatal eating assessment tool: development and content validation. *Neonatal Network*, *36*(6), 359-367.

Pados, B. F., Thoyre, S. M., Knafl, G. J., & Nix, W. B. (2017). Heart rate variability as a feeding intervention outcome measure in the preterm infant. *Advances in neonatal care: official journal of the National Association of Neonatal Nurses*, *17*(5), E10.

Palmer, M. M., Crawley, K., & Blanco, I. (1993). NOMAS: nutritive suck: tongue. *J Perinatol*.

Palmquist, A. E., Holdren, S. M., & Fair, C. D. (2020). "It was all taken away": Lactation, embodiment, and resistance among mothers caring for their very-low-birth-weight infants in the neonatal intensive care unit. *Social Science & Medicine*, *244*, 112648.

Park, J., Pados, B. F., & Thoyre, S. M. (2018). Systematic review: What is the evidence for the side-lying position for feeding preterm infants? *Advances in Neonatal Care*, *18*(4), 285-294.

Parker, L. A., Sullivan, S., Krueger, C., Kelechi, T., & Mueller, M. (2012). Effect of early breast milk expression on milk volume and timing of lactogenesis stage II among mothers of very low birth weight infants: a pilot study. *Journal of Perinatology, 32*(3), 205-209.

Pawling, R., Cannon, P. R., McGlone, F. P., & Walker, S. C. (2017). C-tactile afferent stimulating touch carries a positive affective value. *PloS One, 12*(3), e0173457.

Pelentsov, L. J., Laws, T. A., & Esterman, A. J. (2015). The supportive care needs of parents caring for a child with a rare disease: a scoping review. *Disability and Health Journal, 8*(4), 475-491.

Penny, F., Judge, M., Brownell, E., McGrath, J. M., & Gephart, S. (2018). What is the evidence for use of a supplemental feeding tube device as an alternative supplemental feeding method for breastfed infants? *Advances in Neonatal Care, 18*(1), 31-37.

Penny, F., Judge, M., Brownell, E. A., & McGrath, J. M. (2019). International Board Certified Lactation Consultants' Practices Regarding Supplemental Feeding Methods for Breastfed Infants. *Journal of Human Lactation, 35*(4), 683-694.

Pérez-Escamilla, R., Martinez, J. L., & Segura-Pérez, S. (2016). Impact of the Baby-friendly Hospital Initiative on breastfeeding and child health outcomes: a systematic review. *Maternal & Child Nutrition, 12*(3), 402-417.

Platt, H. (1962). The Platt Report. *British Medical Journal, 2*(5263), 1341-2.

Prisco, A., Capalbo, D., Guarino, S., Del Giudice, E. M., & Marzuillo, P. (2020). How to interpret symptoms, signs and investigations of dehydration in children with gastroenteritis. *Archives of Disease in Childhood-Education and Practice*.

Quandt, Z. E., Salmeen, K. E., & Block-Kurbisch, I. J. (2020). Thyroid Disorders During Pregnancy, Postpartum, and Lactation. *Maternal-Fetal and Neonatal Endocrinology*, 287-315.

Quigley, M., Embleton, N. D., & McGuire, W. (2019). Formula versus donor breast milk for feeding preterm or low birth weight infants. *Cochrane Database of Systematic Reviews*, (7).

Quigley, M. A., Kelly, Y. J., & Sacker, A. (2009). Infant feeding, solid foods and hospitalisation in the first 8 months after birth. *Archives of Disease in Childhood, 94*(2), 148-150.

Ramsay, D. T., Kent, J. C., Hartmann, R. A., & Hartmann, P. E. (2005). Anatomy of the lactating human breast redefined with ultrasound imaging. *Journal of Anatomy, 206*(6), 525-534.

Regan, S., & Brown, A. (2019). Experiences of online breastfeeding support: Support and reassurance versus judgement and misinformation. *Maternal & Child Nutrition, 15*(4), e12874.

Reimers, P., Shenker, N., Weaver, G., & Coutsoudis, A. (2018). Using donor human milk to feed vulnerable term infants: a case series in KwaZulu Natal, South Africa. *International Breastfeeding Journal, 13*(1), 1-8.

Rempel, G. R., Ravindran, V., Rogers, L. G., & Magill-Evans, J. (2013). Parenting under pressure: A grounded theory of parenting young children with life-threatening congenital heart disease. *Journal of Advanced Nursing, 69*(3), 619-630.

Reynolds et al. (2016). Fiberoptic endoscopic evaluation of swallowing. *Advances in Neonatal Care, 16*(1), 37-43.

Riskin, A., Almog, M., Peri, R., Halasz, K., Srugo, I., & Kessel, A. (2012). Changes in immunomodulatory constituents of human milk in response to active infection in the nursing infant. *Pediatric Research, 71*(2), 220-225.

Riva, E., Agostoni, C., Biasucci, G., Trojan, S., Luotti, D., Fiori, L., & Giovannini, M. (1996). Early breastfeeding is linked to higher intelligence quotient scores in dietary treated phenylketonuric children. *Acta Paediatrica, 85*(1), 56-58.

Rodriguez, E. M., Dunn, M. J., Zuckerman, T., Vannatta, K., Gerhardt, C. A., & Compas, B. E. (2012). Cancer-related sources of stress for children with cancer and their parents. *Journal of Pediatric Psychology, 37*(2), 185-197.

Rodriguez, N. A., Miracle, D. J., & Meier, P. P. (2005). Sharing the science on human milk feedings with mothers of very-low-birth-weight infants. *Journal of Obstetric, Gynecologic, & Neonatal Nursing, 34*(1), 109-119.

Rollins, N. C., Bhandari, N., Hajeebhoy, N., Horton, S., Lutter, C. K., Martines, J. C., ... & Group, T. L. B. S. (2016). Why invest, and what it will take to improve breastfeeding practices? *The Lancet*, *387*(10017), 491-504.

Rosenberg, J., Amaral, J. G., Sklar, C. M., Connolly, B. L., Temple, M. J., John, P., & Chait, P. G. (2008). Gastrostomy and gastrojejunostomy tube placements: outcomes in children with gastroschisis, omphalocele, and congenital diaphragmatic hernia. *Radiology*, *248*(1), 247-253.

Rudra, S., Adibe, O. O., Malcolm, W. F., Smith, P. B., Cotten, C. M., & Greenberg, R. G. (2016). Gastrostomy tube placement in infants with congenital diaphragmatic hernia: Frequency, predictors, and growth outcomes. *Early Human Development*, *103*, 97-100.

Sachdeva, M., Murki, S., Oleti, T. P., & Kandraju, H. (2015). Intermittent versus continuous phototherapy for the treatment of neonatal non-hemolytic moderate hyperbilirubinemia in infants more than 34 weeks of gestational age: a randomized controlled trial. *European Journal of Pediatrics*, *174*(2), 177-181.

Salim, N., Shabani, J., Peven, K., Rahman, Q. S. U., Kc, A., Shamba, D., ... & Lawn, J. E. (2021). Kangaroo mother care: EN-BIRTH multi-country validation study. *BMC Pregnancy and Childbirth*, *21*(1), 1-16.

Sarki, M., Parlesak, A., & Robertson, A. (2019). Comparison of national cross-sectional breast-feeding surveys by maternal education in Europe (2006–2016). *Public Health Nutrition*, *22*(5), 848-861.

Savenije, O. E., & Brand, P. L. (2006). Accuracy and precision of test weighing to assess milk intake in newborn infants. *Archives of Disease in Childhood-Fetal and Neonatal Edition*, *91*(5), F330-F332.

Scott, J. A., & Colin, W. B. (2002). Breastfeeding: reasons for starting, reasons for stopping and problems along the way. *Breastfeeding Review*, *10*(2), 13.

Shah, V., Taddio, A., McMurtry, C. M., Halperin, S. A., Noel, M., Riddell, R. P., & Chambers, C. T. (2015). Pharmacological and combined interventions to reduce vaccine injection pain in children and adults: Systematic review and meta-analysis. *The Clinical Journal of Pain*.

Shaker, C. S. (2017, April). Infant-guided, co-regulated feeding in the neonatal intensive care unit. Part II: interventions to promote neuroprotection and safety. In *Seminars in Speech and Language* (Vol. 38, No. 02, pp. 106-115). Thieme Medical Publishers.

Shields, L., Zhou, H., Pratt, J., Taylor, M., Hunter, J., & Pascoe, E. (2012). Family-centred care for hospitalised children aged 0-12 years. *Cochrane Database of Systematic Reviews*, (10).

Shukla, C., & Basheer, R. (2016). Metabolic signals in sleep regulation: recent insights. *Nature and Science of Sleep*, *8*, 9-21.

Simpson, D. A., Carson, C., Kurinczuk, J. J., & Quigley, M. A. (2021). Trends and inequalities in breastfeeding continuation from 1 to 6 weeks: findings from six population-based British cohorts, 1985–2010. *European Journal of Clinical Nutrition*, 1-9.

Simpson, D. A., Quigley, M. A., Kurinczuk, J. J., & Carson, C. (2019). Twenty-five-year trends in breastfeeding initiation: The effects of sociodemographic changes in Great Britain, 1985-2010. *PloS One*, *14*(1), e0210838.

Smith, J., Cheater, F., & Bekker, H. (2015). Parents' experiences of living with a child with a long-term condition: a rapid structured review of the literature. *Health Expectations*, *18*(4), 452-474.

Smith, P. H. (2018). Social justice at the core of breastfeeding protection, promotion and support: a conceptualization. *Journal of Human Lactation*, *34*(2), 220-225.

Smolina, K., Morgan, S. G., Hanley, G. E., Oberlander, T. F., & Mintzes, B. (2016). Postpartum domperidone use in British Columbia: a retrospective cohort study. *CMAJ Open*, *4*(1), E13.

Smolina, K., Mintzes, B., Hanley, G. E., Oberlander, T. F., & Morgan, S. G. (2016). The association between domperidone and ventricular arrhythmia in the postpartum period. *Pharmacoepidemiology and Drug Safety*, *25*(10), 1210-1214.

Sneyers, B., Duceppe, M. A., Frenette, A. J., Burry, L. D., Rico, P., Lavoie, A., ... & Perreault, M. M. (2020). Strategies for the prevention and treatment of iatrogenic withdrawal from opioids and benzodiazepines in critically ill neonates, children and adults: a systematic review of clinical studies. *Drugs*, *80*(12), 1211-1233.

Sooben, R. D. (2012). Breastfeeding patterns in infants with Down's syndrome: A literature review. *British Journal of Midwifery*, 20(3), 187-192.

Spangler, A., & Wambach, K. (2014). *Clinical Guidelines for the Establishment of Exclusive Breastfeeding.* International Lactation Consultant Association.

Spitz, R. A. (1945). Hospitalism: An inquiry into the genesis of psychiatric conditions in early childhood. In 0. Fenichel. *The Psychoanalytic Study of the Child. Vol, 1.*

Spitz, R. A., & Wolf, K. M. (1946). Anaclitic depression: An inquiry into the genesis of psychiatric conditions in early childhood, II. *The Psychoanalytic Study of the Child*, 2(1), 313-342.

Steele, C. (2018). Best practices for handling and administration of expressed human milk and donor human milk for hospitalized preterm infants. *Frontiers in Nutrition*, 76.

Stuebe, A. (2009). The risks of not breastfeeding for mothers and infants. *Reviews in Obstetrics and Gynecology*, 2(4), 222.

Stuebe, A. (2015). Associations between lactation, maternal carbohydrate metabolism, and cardiovascular health. *Clinical Obstetrics and Gynecology*, 58(4), 827.

Sutherland, T., Pierce, C. B., Blomquist, J. L., & Handa, V. L. (2012). Breastfeeding practices among first-time mothers and across multiple pregnancies. *Maternal and Child Health Journal*, 16(8), 1665-1671.

Terp, K., Weis, J., & Lundqvist, P. (2021). Parents' Views of Family-Centered Care at a Pediatric Intensive Care Unit—A Qualitative Study. *Frontiers in Pediatrics*, 9, 725040.

Thomas, J., Marinelli, K. A., & Academy of Breastfeeding Medicine. (2016). ABM Clinical Protocol# 16: Breastfeeding the Hypotonic Infant, Revision 2016. *Breastfeeding Medicine*, 11(6), 271-276.

Thomas, V. Breastfeeding Sick Babies. In Brown, A., & Jones, W. (Eds.). (2019). *A Guide to Supporting Breastfeeding for the Medical Profession.* Routledge.

Thomson, J., Shah, S. S., Simmons, J. M., Sauers-Ford, H. S., Brunswick, S., Hall, D., ... & Beck, A. F. (2016). Financial and social hardships in families of children with medical complexity. *The Journal of Pediatrics*, *172*, 187-193.

Thomson, G., & Trickey, H. (2013). What works for breastfeeding peer support-time to get real. *European Medical Journal: Gynaecology and Obstetrics*, *2013*(1), 15-22.

Torowicz, D. L., Seelhorst, A., Froh, E. B., & Spatz, D. L. (2015). Human milk and breastfeeding outcomes in infants with congenital heart disease. *Breastfeeding Medicine*, *10*(1), 31-37.

Trickey, H., Thomson, G., Grant, A., Sanders, J., Mann, M., Murphy, S., & Paranjothy, S. (2018). A realist review of one-to-one breastfeeding peer support experiments conducted in developed country settings. *Maternal & Child Nutrition*, *14*(1), e12559.

Vanguri, S., Rogers-McQuade, H., Sriraman, N. K., & Academy of Breastfeeding Medicine. (2021). ABM Clinical Protocol# 14: Breastfeeding-Friendly Physician's Office—Optimizing Care for Infants and Children. *Breastfeeding Medicine*, *16*(3), 175-184.

van Oers, H. A., Haverman, L., Limperg, P. F., van Dijk-Lokkart, E. M., Maurice-Stam, H., & Grootenhuis, M. A. (2014). Anxiety and depression in mothers and fathers of a chronically ill child. *Maternal and Child Health Journal*, *18*(8), 1993-2002.

Ventura, A. K. (2017). Associations between breastfeeding and maternal responsiveness: a systematic review of the literature. *Advances in Nutrition*, *8*(3), 495-510.

Verstraete, S., Verbruggen, S. C., Hordijk, J. A., Vanhorebeek, I., Dulfer, K., Güiza, F., ... & Van den Berghe, G. (2019). Long-term developmental effects of withholding parenteral nutrition for 1 week in the paediatric intensive care unit: a 2-year follow-up of the PEPaNIC international, randomised, controlled trial. *The Lancet Respiratory Medicine*, *7*(2), 141-153.

Victora, C. G., Bahl, R., Barros, A. J., França, G. V., Horton, S., Krasevec, J., ... & Group, T. L. B. S. (2016). Breastfeeding in the 21st century: epidemiology, mechanisms, and lifelong effect. *The Lancet*, *387*(10017), 475-490.

Vonneilich, N., Lüdecke, D., & Kofahl, C. (2016). The impact of care on family and health-related quality of life of parents with chronically ill and disabled children. *Disability and Rehabilitation*, *38*(8), 761-767.

Walker, M. (2008). Breastfeeding the late preterm infant. *Journal of Obstetric, Gynecologic & Neonatal Nursing, 37*(6), 692-701.

Walker, M. (2021). *Breastfeeding Management for the Clinician: Using the Evidence*. Jones & Bartlett Learning.

Wambach, K., & Spencer, B. (2021). *Breastfeeding and Human Lactation.* Jones & Bartlett Learning.

Weaver, G., Bertino, E., Gebauer, C., Grovslien, A., Mileusnic-Milenovic, R., Arslanoglu, S., ... & Picaud, J. C. (2019). Recommendations for the establishment and operation of human milk banks in Europe: a consensus statement from the European Milk Bank Association (EMBA). *Frontiers in Pediatrics, 7*, 53.

West, D. D. L., & Marasco, L. (2009). *Breastfeeding Mother's Guide to Making More Milk*. McGraw-Hill.

Wikström, B. M. (2001). Works of art: a complement to theoretical knowledge when teaching nursing care. *Journal of Clinical Nursing, 10*(1), 25-32.

Willette et al., (2016). Fiberoptic examination of swallowing in the breastfeeding infant. *The Laryngoscope, 126*(7), 1681-1686.

Wolf & Glass. (1992). Feeding and Swallowing Disorders in Infancy: Assessment and Management. Hammill Institute on Disabilities, USA.

Woolf, C., Muscara, F., Anderson, V. A., & McCarthy, M. C. (2016). Early traumatic stress responses in parents following a serious illness in their child: A systematic review. *Journal of Clinical Psychology in Medical Settings, 23*(1), 53-66.

World Health Organization. (2014). *Comprehensive implementation plan on maternal, infant and young child nutrition* (No. WHO/NMH/NHD/14.1). World Health Organization.

World Health Organization. (2018). Implementation guidance: protecting, promoting and supporting breastfeeding in facilities providing maternity and newborn services: the revised baby-friendly hospital initiative. Available at: https://apps.who.int/iris/bitstream/handle/10665/272943/9789241513807-eng.pdf

World Health Organization. (1981). *International Code of Marketing of Breast-milk Substitutes*. World Health Organization.

Yang, R., Chen, D., Deng, Q., & Xu, X. (2020). The effect of donor human milk on the length of hospital stay in very low birthweight infants: a systematic review and meta-analysis. *International Breastfeeding Journal*, 15(1), 1-10.

Yang, W. C., Zhao, L. L., Li, Y. C., Chen, C. H., Chang, Y. J., Fu, Y. C., & Wu, H. P. (2013). Bodyweight loss in predicting neonatal hyperbilirubinemia 72 hours after birth in term newborn infants. *BMC Pediatrics*, 13(1), 1-7.

Young, J., McCann, D., Watson, K., Pitcher, A., Bundy, R., & Greathead, D. (2006). Negotiation of care for a hospitalised child: nursing perspectives. *Neonatal, Paediatric & Child Health Nursing*, 9(3).

Zazulak, J., Sanaee, M., Frolic, A., Knibb, N., Tesluk, E., Hughes, E., & Grierson, L. E. (2017). The art of medicine: arts-based training in observation and mindfulness for fostering the empathic response in medical residents. *Medical Humanities*, 43(3), 192-198.

Zhang, F., Cheng, J., Yan, S., Wu, H., & Bai, T. (2019). Early feeding behaviors and breastfeeding outcomes after cesarean section. *Breastfeeding Medicine*, 14(5), 325-333.

Zhang, Z., Zhu, Y., Zhang, L., & Wan, H. (2018). What factors influence exclusive breastfeeding based on the theory of planned behaviour. *Midwifery*, 62, 177-182.

Zimman, L. (2017). Transgender language reform: Some challenges and strategies for promoting trans-affirming, gender-inclusive language. *Journal of Language and Discrimination*, 1(1), 83-104.

Index

H

Hands off approach 36, 40

Hands on pumping 158, 163

Health Visitor (HV) 12, 36, 51

High Dependency Unit (HDU) 112, 251, 266

High calorie need 21, 77, 94, 118, 211, 213

High Flow Nasal Cannula (HFNC) 68, 78, 201

High-Frequency Oscillatory Ventilation (HFOV) 81

Hindmilk 192

Hospital bag 245

Hostility 99-100

Human milk oligosaccharides (HMOs) 25, 30

Hypernatraemia 66

Hypertonia 77, 197

Hypoglycaemia 107, 167, 170, 181, 205, 216, 272

Hypotonia 21, 57, 68, 77, 117, 120, 204, 210-1, 213, 217, 219, 282

Hypoxic Ischaemic Encephalopathy (HIE) 82

I-K

Iatrogenic

  breastfeeding modification 78, 111

  complication 195

  infection 32

  withdrawal 197-8, 224

Immune system 25, 29, 97, 163, 170

Immunoglobulins 25, 30, 96, 163, 193, 202-3, 220, 259

Immunocompromised 63, 97, 159-60, 193, 220

Inclusive language 17

International Board Certified Lactation Consultant (IBCLC) 12, 18, 20, 70, 79, 81, 84-5, 105-8, 110, 158, 164, 167, 173, 191, 222, 264, 279

Intravenous (IV) 58, 180, 210, 221, 254

Jaundice 10, 42, 57, 65-6, 71, 87-8, 107, 171, 181, 217

Made in the USA
Coppell, TX
25 June 2024

33910320R00184